Why Dialogue Does Cure

Jaakko Seikkula

Why Dialogue Does Cure

Explaining What Makes Dialogue Unprecedentedly Effective in Difficult Crises

Springer

Jaakko Seikkula
Department of Psychology
University of Jyväskylä
Jyväskylä, Finland

ISBN 978-3-031-91293-1 ISBN 978-3-031-91294-8 (eBook)
https://doi.org/10.1007/978-3-031-91294-8

This Springer imprint is published by the registered company Springer Nature Switzerland AG
The registered company address is: Gewerbestrasse 11, 6330 Cham, Switzerland

Preface: Dialogue Does Cure: But Why?

"These results cannot be true." "We here do not believe in the results of Open Dialogue in Western Lapland and that practice is not possible here." You often hear comments like this in psychiatry. In dialogical practice it is possible to achieve a recovery that cannot be imagined in conventional psychiatry. Over the last couple of decades, the distance between the humanistic dialogical approach and conventional treatment has only increased. The aim of this book is to shorten this distance by describing in a concise way why dialogical practice can be so effective. My aim is also to reiterate some of the findings to clarify that a different kind of practice is indeed possible.

The idea for this book came to life at the height of the pandemic. With mobility restrictions, there was plenty of time to reflect on my experiences over 45 years of working in and researching mental health services. This period has been very rich in many ways. For me it has meant the opportunity to do what I have wanted to do. Throughout my career, I have wanted to work with mental health crises, especially the most difficult problems. This was already a theme in my studies at the University of Jyväskylä. The topic of my master's thesis in psychology was risk factors for adult mental health problems in preschool age. I focused (the study was a collaboration among five students) on risk factors that predict psychotic problems. This work was so fascinating that, upon graduation, I immediately went into clinical work in psychiatry.

And that's the path I've been on all my professional life. First, I worked as a clinical psychologist, the longest at Keropudas Hospital in Western Lapland. After moving to the University of Jyväskylä in 1998, my research focus remained on the development of systems of care for severe mental health crises, and especially on understanding dialogue as a part of it. I thus have a relatively long perspective on the development of mental health care in Finland and worldwide. I am a family therapist, and working with families has been a central part of my interest. Without the involvement of families, an adequate level of care cannot be provided. In my home country, Finland, there are good opportunities for psychotherapy and family therapy within the public system.

We developed family-centered care with enthusiasm in the 1980s. At that time, there were many different psychotherapies and competition between them. There was a lot of interest in understanding human beings and everyone wanted training. In the early 1990s, there was huge enthusiasm among those interested in psychotherapy to develop the system of care. I was very interested in language-oriented psychotherapeutic methods and related social constructionism. In short, the idea was that reality is constructed in our descriptions; that is, people's problems are only defined as problems if we define them as such in our conversation. There are no problems that are objectively the same everywhere.

But then everything changed. At the beginning of the 1990s, Evidence-Based Medicine entered the field of mental health and, with it, treatment of excellence guidelines for different diagnostic categories. The rationale for these guidelines was that research into the causes and treatment of various problems was growing so rapidly that it was important to create some system for systematizing scientific knowledge to develop treatment. So, it is a very good principle. But a coup d'état took place, which resulted in research being very poorly tailored to the actual treatment situation. The guidelines for treatment, in Finland called "Current Care Recommendations," defined right and wrong scientific evidence. It became standard to emphasize that the highest level of evidence for a particular treatment method is provided by double-blind trials. This means that in the same population—for example, among people living in the same town—patients who need treatment are randomly assigned to a group receiving a particular treatment (the study group) and a comparable group not receiving treatment (the control group). The results of the treatment are assessed by measuring the change in symptoms at baseline and during follow-up in both groups. Since all other factors influencing treatment had to be controlled to ensure comparability between the groups, the system began to emphasize very simple treatment methods and their measurement.

Therapy methods based on psychotherapeutic encounter and an understanding of the whole person are very difficult to control and randomize. And it is difficult to monitor their results just by measuring simple symptoms. Psychotherapists made frequent reference to such research, which was very unfortunate, because the field of mental health care has almost entirely fallen victim to the data generated by studies that are one-sided and simplify people's problems. The preference for randomized trials also began to produce explanations of problems in a very straightforward way. At the same time as new brain research methods were being developed, research into the causes of problems increasingly focused on brain research, because that was believed to provide the most valid and stable information. In the 1990s, the idea that the cause of human activity could be reduced to brain function and that human problems such as schizophrenia and depression could be reduced to some problem of brain function or structure or genes became widespread. Some extremists began to talk about schizophrenia being a brain disease. Others might say that depression is caused by a neurological imbalance. Others argued that psychotic behavior is neurotoxic and therefore the most important treatment is to medicate the brain immediately. All these were speculations without sufficient scientific evidence.

The increasing popularity of brain scans as such did not cause any of these changes. Studying the brain and the nervous system is very important for the development of psychological knowledge. It is more a question of the fact that those who do not pay attention to the complexity of the phenomenon began to make gross simplifications of the results of brain studies. And those who wanted humane psychotherapeutic treatment did not have the scientific evidence to offer better information. We did lose this competition. The enthusiasm of the early 1990s has turned into anguish leaving no room for human encounter in psychiatric care.

I have been very fortunate to have been involved in the development and research of Open Dialogue, originally developed in the Finnish Western Lapland. It is based on strong scientific evidence, where people in need are treated as full human beings in their own network. The results have been staggering on almost all measures. I believe this is linked to the concept of dialogue, where listening to and accepting the other is central. But every year it seems harder and harder to say what dialogue is and how it helps. It is as if the distance between mainstream psychiatry and the dialogical approach based on human encounter has grown so long that one can no longer hear the other.

So, I decided to write this book. My idea is to summarize the core elements for a system of care that does not focus on eliminating the symptoms of the one in need of help, but on meeting the full human. All the phenomena described in this book have developed in collaboration with very creative people: first in Tornio with the inspiring team. In particular, I would like to mention my collaboration with the chief psychiatrists Birgitta Alakare and Jyrki Keränen. Also crucial was the cooperation with psychologists Kauko Haarakangas and Markku Sutela. We were in the same family therapy training in the early 1980s. The memory of Birgitta, Kauko, and Markku lives on in my work every day. In addition to them, I should really mention all my colleagues, because it was a shared experience to work at Keropudas Hospital. It made me richer as a person and as a therapist. I am grateful that my collaboration and friendship with psychologist Tapio Salo continues. Tapio's contribution is great in the way he approaches dialogical therapy as an individual psychodynamic psychotherapist, thus enriching the polyphony of the dialogical approach.

My work in the university has also allowed me to focus on the essentials. The cooperation with my teacher and mentor, Professor Jukka Aaltonen, has been important over the decades. I have been very fortunate in the sense that our experience of dialogical work and open dialogues has started to attract growing interest internationally. I have made friends with people who are fundamentally deepening my knowledge and skills. Most important was the long-standing collaboration with Professor Tom Andersen of the University of Tromsø. This collaboration ended with his death in 2007, but in a way, Tom is always with me as an inner voice.

The crystallization of dialogicity into an understandable presentation would not have been possible without a long collaboration with Professor Tom Erik Arnkil. Tom has brought social insight and a philosophical perspective with his deep knowledge of life.

Dialogue is always personal. I engage in dialogue as a human being, even if I am carrying out a professional task. Therefore, we cannot fail to mention the importance of personal relationships. I have talked a lot about love as the embodiment of dialogue. My dearest daughters Aura and Heta and their families have changed me more than anything else in my life. The love of my wife Sofia and the collaboration in dialogical therapy and education in Open Dialogue that has intensified in recent years are my life source.

Thanks to Kuva ja Mieli for publishing my book in Finnish. Publishing such a book is always a cultural achievement. No great financial gains are expected. I am also extremely grateful to Springer Verlag for publishing the book in English. This would not have been possible without the huge work of Alita Taylor and Mark Hopfenbeck, who took care of the revision of English language. The most important thing is to keep the flame of humanism alive, even if people are threatened by fragmenting treatment methods and the pathologizing of problems from all sides.

Helsinki, Finland Jaakko Seikkula
May 2025

Contents

Chapter 1
Dialogical Forms of Practice and Open Dialogues

Dialogue is an inevitable part of life. It happens in every human encounter—in the family, among friends, in the classroom, when dealing with authorities, at the doctor's office, or in psychotherapy. Dialogue also takes place in all forms of client work, because without dialogue with their clients, professionals cannot understand their situation. In general, we understand dialogue as a way of exchange that allows us to learn about each other in all kinds of interactions. So, it is not special to talk about dialogue in therapy, because it is also an element of all forms of helping others. Dailogue is seen a means to an end: If we communicate well with the other person, we understand them better.

However, this book describes dialogue from a different perspective, as a fundamental dimension of life, rather than as a means of discussion. Dialogue is not a means to improve interaction or to achieve a particular goal, but is a value in and of itself. Dialogue is life, and it can manifest itself as a value in itself in a wide variety of situations. I know of school classes where work is organized in a dialogical way. I have visited companies where developing dialogue is a key factor in the development of cooperation between employees. In some areas, social workers have adopted dialogue as a key principle while organizing their work. One cardiologist told me that his work had changed fundamentally since he adopted the processes of dialogue as part of his work. A wide range of different forms of dialogical assistance has emerged in the context of psychological encounters, ranging from individual psychotherapy (Hermans, 2004; Leiman, 2004; Lysaker & Lysaker, 2004; Stiles et al., 2004), family therapy (Andersen, 1991; Anderson, 1997; Anderson & Goolishian, 1988; Rober, 2017; Seikkula & Arnkil, 2014), and to group therapy (Sempere & Fuenzalida, 2017). Tom Erik Arnkil and his team have developed a specific dialogical way of working with social networks in problematic situations (Seikkula & Arnkil, 2014). They have named this dialogical work "anticipation dialogues" and "early discussion of worries." This innovation is very interesting because it is not based on psychotherapy but on the dilemmas with and among multidisciplinary social networks. A dialogical approach can therefore be developed in a very wide range of interactional situations.

J. Seikkula, *Why Dialogue Does Cure*,
https://doi.org/10.1007/978-3-031-91294-8_1

In this opening chapter, I will review the basic concepts of dialogicity, the practical basics of dialogical aid work, and the starting points of Open Dialogue, so that the reader knows what we are talking about when we talk about dialogical aid work.

No More Helper and Helpee, but a Shared Experience

Dialogical working methods bring a new perspective to psychological help. Whereas traditional methods of helping are based on work led by therapists or other facilitators who apply interventions specific to each method to address clients' problems, in dialogical work, clients take the lead. The aim is not to change clients, for example, by eliminating their symptoms, but to create a shared experience by opening up to new perspectives. *The processes follow clients' stories about their lives and problems, and professionals (teachers, doctors, social workers, nurses, work community consultants, and psychotherapists) are involved in building a new shared experience by responding to clients' expressions.* The success of the process is reflected in the way in which the facilitator, in his or her own response, manages to respect the client's point of view, enabling them to better understand their own experience and, thus, to find new resources for managing their lives and becoming the author of their own life story.

In this book, I focus extensively on dialogicity and on a particular Open Dialogue mindset for helping those in need dealing with the most difficult crises. Although it is indeed psychotherapeutic helping, there are many benefits to adopting dialogicity in all kinds of encounters. As a psychotherapist, my examples often come from the most difficult crises in psychotherapeutic situations. My area of expertise is family therapy and the application of family therapy to life-threatening psychological crises where dialogue has shown its power. Nonetheless, a dialogical approach can be applied just as successfully with one person.

Dialogue became important when psychotherapies began to emphasize the centrality of language: how we make sense of our life experiences and problems in conversation. In my work, this shift began in the 1980s. After my own training as a family therapist had taught me to view the family as a unit in which different family members construct the family system through their behavior, the linguistic shift focused attention on the different family members' accounts of their own family and its problems. This perspective was first introduced by solution-focused therapists (Furman & Ahola, 2020; Kim Berg, 2001), who drew attention to the fact that the speech that defines the problem is, in fact, the problem, rather than a behavior or a symptom per se. Around the same time, Michael White and David Epston (White & Epston, 1990) developed narrative therapy, working specifically with families with children. They emphasized that people create their lives in their unique narratives. Good therapy comes from being interested in all the narratives and no longer trying to define one family system or family problem. Harry Goolishian and Harlene Anderson were the first to call family therapy a dialogue (Anderson & Goolishian, 1988). The decisive change to open up family therapy as a shared process was made by the Norwegian psychiatrist Tom Andersen, who, with his team, developed the idea of the reflective team (Andersen, 1991; Andersen, 2022). The revolutionary dimension of the reflective team was that therapists now openly shared, in front of the family, what they thought about what family members were saying. In this way, the therapists' different views became part of a spectrum of different accounts of the problem presented by the family.

In the realm of individual psychotherapy, a dialogical approach began to develop in the context of both cognitive therapy and psychodynamic therapy. In cognitive therapy, Hermans (2004) worked on the concept of internal schemas in the client, saying that schemas are not fixed strategies for action, but represent different voices of the individual's experience. It is not possible to achieve a single fixed perspective or attitude, but the person's experience emerges in each situation and conversation according to the voices that emerge in it. He developed a specific description of the human being as a dialogical self—the Dialogical Self. The psychological reality of inner voices has also been developed by Stiles et al. (2004), stating that "the voices of the mind are memory traces that are activated in new experiences when these experiences resemble in some way the original experience" (p. 92).

Also in individual psychotherapy, the dialogical approach has been developed by Leiman (2004), who integrates constructivist and psychodynamic therapy in a specific Cognitive Analytic Therapy. Stern (2004) also created a new form of psychodynamic therapy, which follows the basic idea of dialogical psychotherapy: to follow the client's story without leading and to participate in it with the therapist's answers without a specific interpretation of the meaning of what the client is telling. He does not call his therapy dialogical, but that is what it is if we follow that definition of dialogicity above. Clients share their dilemmas while therapists, through their responses, respect their own unconditional experiences without steering the client's narrative in any particular direction and interpreting it.

Therapy Meeting Paves the Way for Dialogue, Open Dialogues

My way of working began to develop in a dialogical direction when I worked as a psychologist at the Keropudas Psychiatric Hospital in Tornio beginning in the early 1980s. The common goal of our team was to develop family-centered care so that the families of patients in the hospital would have a greater role in the care of the family member who came to the hospital. Initially, we applied systemic family therapy, but only a very small proportion of families could participate in treatment. The way we worked changed dramatically in 1984 when we started to organize open therapy meetings. Encouraged by an innovation originally developed in Turku by Professor Yrjö Alanen's team, we changed the treatment practice so that the treatment team no longer discussed treatment or treatment plans without the patient but decided to always include the patient in all discussions concerning him or her. Absolute openness is a revolutionary dimension of the therapy meeting. Everything is done openly from the start so that the care team does not meet first without the patient or his family to plan the discussion. At the same time, we changed our practice so that we always started to invite the patient's family to these joint therapy meetings, where everything was discussed openly in the presence of everyone. The family was therefore no longer invited to family therapy on the basis of some interaction problem we had identified. Instead, familie were automatically invited in all situations. The openness of the therapy meeting was very close to the idea of a reflective team created by Tom Andersen and his colleagues because the thoughts and conclusions of the clinicians were now openly shared.

We received encouraging results from the open therapy meetings. New perspectives on difficult situations emerged and clients[1] developed new solutions to their problems. At the same time, we also had some confusing, unexpected experiences, which forced us to reflect on the rationale for a new open way of working. Whereas in traditional psychiatric care, we were used to defining the problem as precisely as possible and setting treatment goals and the treatment interventions needed to achieve them, we could now find ourselves in dead-end situations where change started with *our* change, not with the clients' change.

There were countless such situations. On one occasion, Antti was admitted to the hospital as a result of excessive alcohol consumption and was psychotic. We met him and his wife the day he arrived at the hospital. The wife told us that she had become so afraid of Antti that she didn't know whether she would dare take him home again. In the ward, Antti's psychosis quickly subsided and after about a week of treatment, we planned for him to go home for a weekend break. However, his wife did not agree to this. After a few weeks, the ward team was very frustrated because the wife did not agree to Antti's return home, even though we felt that Antti had fully recovered. We arranged a therapy meeting, to which the wife came with her mother. When the ward doctor suggested at the meeting that it would be a good idea for Antti to go home on holiday, Antti suddenly stood up and, swearing, threatened his wife with harsh words. We were so convinced of our own treatment plan that we suggested the same thing a second and third time, and each time Antti got angry and threatened his wife. When this happened the third time, fortunately, one of the mental health nurses—thank you, Raija—was sensible enough to start asking us staff what we were doing. Every time we suggested that Antti return home, he started threatening his wife's life. Do we want to have a homicide on our conscience, Raija asked the rest of us. This question made us open our eyes and our stuck thoughts, and we started to reflect on the difficult situation of the family. Obviously, we had not heard the wife's message and had not understood the depth of their crisis.

The change started with our change. This was very confusing because traditionally the goal of treatment is to change the patient and/or their family. Our role was to be a healer who knows what methods to use at any given time to implement the treatment plan. But now we were already in a new paradigm that we did not yet

[1] By client, I refer to all members of your personal social network. So, for example, in a family discussion, the client is not only the one that we call as patient but also the family members.

understand. When we opened the door for the patient and his family to participate in all discussions, they started to actively share their views and to let their voices be heard. Often, they also found new resources for difficult situations. In Antti's case, we agreed together to set aside more time for Antti and his wife to talk together. In these discussions, after a few months, they announced that they could no longer continue together and that they would separate.

In order to understand the new phenomena of care, we were "forced" to start studying unprecedented events and the functioning of the practice of therapy meetings. We began to reflect on the dialogues of the therapy meeting. For Antti, the change started when the carers responded to clients in a new way. At first, we did not talk about dialogues, but afterward, it was easy to see that this was the essence of dialogue: responding to the other person and matching what they say. This basic event helped us to understand the Russian literary scholar and philosopher Mikhail Bakhtin's description of polyphonic and dialogical life. It was only after many years that the new way of working was called Open Dialogue (Aaltonen et al., 2011; Seikkula et al., 1995).

One particular dimension of Open Dialogue is that it encompasses both the planning and the implementation of psychiatric care and psychotherapy. Initially, it was a new way of psychiatric care planning for me and the whole team, but as we were making treatment plans, we found the dialogue itself to be very therapeutic. Often a good treatment planning discussion in open treatment meetings was the best treatment. Over time, new applications of open family discussions in very different contexts also began to develop. I myself moved to the University of Jyväskylä in 1998, where I met clients in a psychotherapy clinic. In therapy, I constantly applied the open working style and the idea of working in teams in different dilemmas. I also extended my research on dialogical processes to different contexts that were no longer directly related to psychiatric treatment planning. This gave rise to a form of dialogical therapy, which I describe in this book.

Dialogue Is Life, and Outside It Is Death

One of the most influential theorists on the basic ideas of dialogical encounter and dialogical therapy is the literary scholar and philosopher Mikhail Bakhtin. Almost all trends in dialogical therapy refer to his dialogical worldview as the basis for his work. His conception of man can be summed up in a couple of quotes from one of his key books, The Problems of Dostoevsky's Poetics (Bakhtin, 1984). He wrote this book twice. The first time was in 1929 when it was a description of the central elements of his new dialogical worldview. The second version of the book appeared in 1963 in a more developed form in Russian and in this book, he opens up in greater depth a new philosophical description of life. Some of his notes have been added to the English edition of the book. In one of them, he sums up his own worldview by stating:

> "Life by its very nature is dialogical. To live means to participate in dialogue; to ask questions, to heed, to respond, to agree, and so forth". *In this dialogue a person participates wholly and throughout his whole life: with his eyes, lips, hands, soul, spirit, with his whole body, and deeds.* He invests his entire self in discourse, and this discourse enters into the dialogical fabric of human life, into the world symposium (Bakhtin, 1984, p. 293).

Bakhtin thus states that dialogue is life. Life is to participate in dialogue with all our actions and with our whole body. All our actions are always in relation to other people and therefore also communication, waiting for a response. It is in this encounter that the self is born. He also says another really radical thing about our view of the world: We participate in dialogue throughout life, from the first breath after birth. I will discuss this in more detail in Chap. 4. Studies of intersubjectivity have identified participation in dialogical response as a central dimension of human psychic life. At birth, we have an innate inherited ability to initiate with body movements, looks, and vocalizations, and to respond to the initiation of others. This biological innate capacity carries us for about the first 6 months of life, after which we begin to learn the voluntary skills of dialogue and communication.

This is a stunning observation. There are really only two basic conditions of life. When we are born, we must learn to breathe. If we don't breathe, we die. In the same way, our first experience is to learn to be in dialogue. If we are not in dialogue, we die. This basic assumption about life is the basis of dialogical therapy. The goal is to create dialogue because, in a dialogical relationship, we get a response when we are heard and accepted. The goal of therapy is to be heard because when one is heard and acknowledged in the response of another, a dialogical reciprocal relationship is created.

Bakhtin defines dialogue as:

> Dialogue here is not the threshold to action, it is the action itself. It is not a means for revealing, for bringing to the surface the already-made character of a person; no, in dialogue a person not only shows himself outwardly, but he becomes for the first time that which he is—and, we repeat, not only for others but for himself as well. To be means to communicate dialogically. (Bakhtin, 1984, p. 252)

He gives an important guideline for psychotherapists: The aim of therapy is to create a dialogue in the here and now, because in a dialogue a person becomes himself for the first time, including both his own experiences of himself and the experiences of others about him. We become ourselves as human beings in our expressions if the other person present receives and responds to them. An expression is not a statement of what I think dressed up as a finished thought, but actually the opposite. Only in the response I receive I know what I feel and think. The response does not have to be a clear comment dressed up in words and sentences, but the other person's response to me is immediate and direct, whether he or she means it or not. For example, the fact that the other person listens to what I am saying without obviously flinching is a response in which I begin to know myself better. With that kind of response, I begin to wonder if I am boring company and if what I have to say is important.

Dialogical understanding is very different from the psychological description of human beings as different personality traits and associated brain structures. These descriptions often aim at permanent descriptions of the human being. Such descriptions have also given rise to a number of psychotherapeutic orientations that provide guidelines for dealing with different personalities and different problems. In dialogical therapy, phenomena are encountered as part of a progressive stream of life, where the most important thing is to understand the meaning of phenomena and people's experiences in the present moment on the basis of the response of the other person.

You Cannot Deny the Truth of the Other

Dialogue is based on the interaction of disconnected individuals and their voices. The only possibility in life is to create a dialogue with others. Bakhtin discovered the fundamental nature of dialogue in his study of the writing style of the classic Russian writers, where his greatest discovery was an understanding of Fyodor Dostoevsky's novel world as very different from that of Leo Tolstoy's, for example. While Tolstoy's novels always have one main character, the hero of the book, Dostoevsky's novels, according to Bakhtin, always have as many main characters as there are characters speaking in the book. The characters in Tolstoy's books complete the story of the book's hero in the way the author wants, whereas in Dostoyevsky's novels, each character has his own truth, which no one else can dispute. So, the only possibility is to try to enter into a dialogue with the other character in order to understand his or her point of view. The characters in the book are in constant dialogue with each other; the books are descriptions of dialogue. In dialogue, the characters in the book begin to understand each other, which is a very challenging situation for the author, because the characters in the book begin to understand each other more than the author does. In their dialogue, a new world is created. The only way for an author to overcome this challenge is to try to enter into a dialogue with his characters. A paradoxical situation arises: The characters in the book are no longer the author's creations to tell the story he wants to tell, but they each create their own reality through dialogue, incorporating all the voices that emerge from that dialogue.

Bakhtin describes this as a polyphonic worldview. We all have our own voices, which are not fixed internal opinions or personality traits but are perspectives on life that are expressed through speech. We live in a multiplicity of voices, where we must seek dialogue with others in order to understand them, and when I understand them, my own understanding of myself changes. Bakhtin says that when we respond to each other, the response becomes our own inner experience; the word becomes inner and is no longer just a means of communication. We are constantly creating reality for others and for ourselves.

It may come as a surprise to the reader that I describe a literary scholar. It was also a great surprise to me when I began to realize that Bakhtin's description of Dostoevsky's literature actually describes very accurately our experiences in open therapy meetings in psychiatric care. As carers, we could not direct and impose the treatment process. The best outcome came from listening to all voices. No one could dispute another's perspective on the problem. When we ourselves changed, the other's change became possible. *This is the essence of a dialogical encounter: How we respond to each other, no longer what change we seek through our questions or interpretations of the patient or family.*

Vertical and Horizontal Polyphony: A New Space of Voices

The speaker's voice is always expressed in dialogue, in relation to other voices. According to Bakhtin, the voice is the speaking consciousness expressed in dialogue (Wertsch, 1991). He states that "one participates in dialogue with one's most essential voice. He participates not only with his thoughts but also with his destiny and all his individuality" (Bakhtin, 1984, p. 293). The self is born in this speech. Experiences expressed in words, in dialogue, become the voice of our lives. The words I utter maybe my own words, or they may also contain the words of other people. Young children already learn polyphonic language at school by reading aloud a text. They read in their own voice but include another voice.

Psychologist Kauko Haarakangas studied the voices of the therapy meeting in his doctoral thesis (Haarakangas, 1997). He made an important distinction about the two-dimensionality of the polyphony of the therapy meeting. Participants in a conversation are having a conversation with each other in a horizontal polyphony. For example, the therapist asks the mother of a family something about her child. When the mother expresses her concern about her teenage daughter being out so late, the two of them are in conversation with each other on a horizontal polyphonic plane. Two voices are involved in this conversation, the therapist's and the mother's. But all dialogues involve other voices, the inner voices of each of the participants themselves. This world of voices is what Kauko Haarakangas called a vertical polyphony with a much richer range of voices. Each listener to the conversation between the therapist and the mother is engaged in his or her own dialogue about the concerns expressed by the mother. Both of them, of course, but also the daughter of concern, her father, and the other clinicians participating in the therapy session.

Everyone participates in an internal vertical dialogue based on their own life experience. In this dialogue, memories may emerge, for example, of a mother's own youth and how her parents dealt with it. The dialogical therapist can invite those voices into the conversation by asking, for example, "If your mother were here now and heard this conversation, what would she say about it? Would she have any advice for this situation?"

For clinicians, this dialogue is very interesting. They are always involved with a certain professional and ethical responsibility. But beyond that, each person also always responds with their own personal voice, which starts to ring out in line with each topic of discussion. Thus, the therapist can be moved if the discussion is about the divorce of the parents if he or she also has experience of his or her own divorce. We can only engage in dialogue as human beings, not as professionals. A psychologist or a doctor will not talk, but Maija and Matti will. In dialogue, we always listen to these different voices, not so much the people who express them. People are always expressed in relation to each other through what they say or otherwise express; they are not ready-made or fixed totalities.

The Uniqueness of Each Situation and the Importance of Responding

When human psychological reality is no longer seen as a set of fixed attributes, our understanding of interactional situations changes. Bakhtin uses the concept of chronotype to describe the fact that each dialogue creates its own unique reality. In other words, reality is created in the moment of encounter, both in conversations and in other forms of communication.

Each social group creates its own social language, which is the basis for the meanings that emerge in each conversation. We contribute to each conversation from a diversity of different groups. I belong to a men's social group, I am of a certain age with shared experiences with people of this age, I am a therapist, I am a university professor, I live in this city, and so on. All these social languages determine my starting point in each conversation. Recognizing the uniqueness of social languages helps to respect and accommodate the specificities of different cultures. For example, people from different national traditions and religions can participate in therapeutic sessions. Respecting the uniqueness of each of these is the basis of a good encounter because everyone needs to experience being heard and respected according to the values of their own social language—their own culture.

But as already said, these only take on meaning in the here-and-now dialogue, where a new reality is always being created. Every conversation is always a first conversation, even if we have met this family ten times before. There is always the possibility of a new understanding. For therapy, this is of great importance. We should not be worried if we repeatedly talk about the same topic, because each time we allow this topic to arise, new meanings will emerge.

I have had the special privilege of participating in open therapy meetings in very different cultures. To my surprise, the dialogue itself can take place in very similar ways in each culture. Respecting and recognizing the uniqueness of the cultures subtly helps the participants to meet, but the dialogical experience itself seems to emerge similarly in China, Japan, the United States, Brazil, Paraguay, Poland, Germany, Spain, Italy, England, and Finland. And in the same way, it can arise with those of different sexual orientations or from different racial backgrounds. Dialogue is universal.

It all comes down to each interaction in the here and now. The basic idea of dialogue is to guarantee an answer to the other. In an oft-repeated phrase, Bakhtin says that there is nothing more terrible for a word (and therefore for a person) than a lack of response. Without a response, what is expressed by the other dies away and naturally affects the expresser's experience of his own word immediately: Is it not significant? Am I not important? Should I express myself violently, for example, to be heard? To be heard is the aim and purpose of interaction. If I am heard, the dialogue has begun. In dialogue, I become the person I am at that moment. The goal is achieved.

What is the response? The response is not so much a piece of information or an explanation of a problem, but rather a sensation of the moment. We respond to each other all the time, even when we are not trying to. When I do not respond to another's initiative, that in itself is a response, whether I want it or not. Bakhtin talks about the immediacy of the response. He says that we recognize each other without the mediation of words and that such a response is, in fact, generated even before we become verbally aware of it. I see myself in your eyes, he might say, or, I borrow your eyes to see myself. The response of the other is therefore an immediate split-second sensation or feeling before the experience is put into words. All this underlines the importance of the way of participating in therapeutic conversations. Interestingly, the philosopher Emmanuel Levinas (Levinas, 1985) also talks about the other waiting for my response. He defines even more precisely that the face of the other awaits my response, and I can never escape this invitation. Everything I do is already an answer, whether I want it or not. Later, I will look in more detail at how we can develop our presence skills as therapists (Chap. 10).

The Importance of Dialogue for Family Meetings

Dialogue is not primarily concerned with what is said, but with how things are said and how they are responded to in a dialogical process (Rober, 2017; Seikkula et al., 1995). The stories told always define the speaker, but what becomes more essential in dialogue is the relationship between the speaker and the interlocutors, reflective partners (Andersen, 1995; Anderson & Goolishian, 1988; White & Epston, 1990). Narratives only come alive in the presence of the listeners and in their response to what is said. In this sense, speaking is a dialogical phenomenon. In therapeutic conversations, however, people in need of therapeutic help do not speak complete narratives but rather broken and incomplete stories. Clients talk about particularly sensitive and emotional experiences, and their stories may be incomplete and contain many contradictions (Gergen, 2009). Clients do not have precise words or phrases to express their sensitive experiences and most pressing concerns. It is this inability to express unambiguously the event or other reason for seeking help that often seems to be the basis for seeking help. Psychological symptoms are a sign that he and his family lack the words to express their most important experiences. Difficult events in their lives in the past have become embedded in the body's memory and are activated as voices of life under the pressures of the moment, but rarely as explicitly told stories. In most cases, only a strong and overwhelming feeling emerges, such as anxiety, panic, depression, or delusions.

Psychotherapy is about finding words for life experiences that are still wordless. In family therapy, in building a new common language, we involve family members as real living and embodied persons. Dialogically, this is very important because, as Mikhail Bakhtin pointed out, the interlocutors are the active co-constructors of the individual's narrative. Each word of a participant in an actual dialogue becomes part of a network of tensions of previously spoken words. Each new word contributes to a topic already started by the one already said. In this process, the thing spoken "cannot fail to be an active participant in a social dialogue" (Bakhtin, 1986, p. 276). Everything said or done is a response to something previously said or done.

Every speaker is the subject of their expression physiologically when they produce their expression with their own body. But only physiologically, because when their expression is heard and seen, it becomes part of the meaning given to it by the responses of all those present. In family therapy, a new language is developed, especially in the responses that family members give to each other in response to the questions and concerns expressed. In addition, therapists have a particular responsibility in that their responses contribute to the construction of a shared experience (Steiner, 1989). We are part of a shared experience in the discussion, which aims to increase understanding of the unique situation of the person in need. This understanding does not come, for example, from giving a diagnosis, but is always based on a shared encounter and sharing of the pain of the client.

Understanding is achieved through an active process, by taking responsibility for responding to the other. In an Open Dialogue, we respond to what has been said in a way that waits for a response from the next speaker. Whether we really hear the other person becomes evident in his or her comments. In a family session, stories unfold gradually and unpredictably from the contradictory and tense influences of all those present. Everything expressed becomes implicitly or explicitly judged by others, and their verbal and non-verbal reactions invite new expressions in a complex dialectical dance of differences and similarities (Baxter, 2004).

Open Dialogues

Open Dialogue is a Finnish innovation developed on the tradition of the need-adapted approach. I describe them here as an example of dialogical practice because Open Dialogue has been researched and provided evidence of the healing power of dialogue—the fundamental question of the book. Later (Chap. 3), I will describe in more detail the emergence of Open Dialogue through the development of the Keropudas Hospital in and around the psychiatric outpatient clinic in Tornio. Here I will describe the outcome of the development process, that is, how dialogicity had evolved by the mid-1990s when we first named the new concept of care "Open Dialogue." As I have already mentioned, its specificity lies in the fact that it is both a way of organizing psychiatric care and a form of dialogical psychotherapy.

The basic idea behind Open Dialogue is very simple. Discussions with the client seeking help, their family, and other social networks are open to all. Nothing about the client's care is discussed without his or her presence. In addition, the basic idea of Open Dialogue is that clinicians work together as a team, participating in all the therapy meetings where the problems that led to the client's need for help are discussed. This simplicity is paradoxical, however, because clinicians give up two "sacred cows": (1) giving up holding discussions about care planning and treatment decisions among staff and (2) giving up interviewing a client or clients by a single clinician and instead starting to conduct, for example, a medical history interview in the presence of the care team. Of course, there are important exceptions to both of these points, but this is the big picture of care delivery. Only by acting in this way can the guiding idea of dialogical therapy be followed, whereby clients lead the clinicians both in the content of the conversation and in the manner of the conversation, and the clinicians' role is to follow them.

Together with Mary Olson and Doug Ziedonis, we developed a document defining an Open Dialogue therapy meeting (Olson et al., 2014), which states that a therapy meeting can be called an Open Dialogue if the following basic elements are met:

1. The discussion is hosted by two or more clinicians.
2. Where possible, the family and social network of the person in need will be involved in the joint process. However, not necessarily all discussions, as dialogue can also take place with a single client.
3. The discussion uses open-ended questions so that clients have the opportunity to talk about what is most important to them at the moment.
4. The discussion is a response to the client's expressions, which is the main thread of the discussion.
5. The dialog will focus on the here-and-now.
6. The dialog is constantly seeking multiple perspectives.
7. The discussion will focus on how things manifest themselves in relationships.
8. The discussion responds to expressions describing problems by accepting them as answers to a difficult life situation. This can be called a normalizing conversation. So, for example, the raging of a family member or the voices of another are seen as normal responses to extreme stress rather than signs of a particular psychopathology.
9. The discussion follows the clients' own words and stories, rather than looking for their symptoms.
10. Open discussion between team members is part of the dialogical process.
11. Team members are transparent in all their discussions, openly explaining their opinions and suggestions.
12. In a dialogue, uncertainty is tolerated, so there is no point in trying to understand the cause of the problem as quickly as possible. Shared dialogical is always more important than conclusions.

Therapy Meeting to Build a Shared Experience

The main forum for Open Dialogue is the therapy meeting, where discussions are not prepared in advance, but everyone enters the room at the same time, sits down, and starts talking. We sit in a circle so that we can see each other. This circle includes the caring team, the person at the center of concern ("the patient"), their family, and possibly other social networks. A similar discussion can also be held with just one patient and the care team.

The conversation does not have a predetermined structure but emerges according to the situation. The discussion starts with an open question to the family and the patient. The aim is to ensure that we start talking to clients about the most topical issue and thus follow what they have to say. Of course, it is good manners to introduce ourselves first and ask some general questions about what everyone is talking about. Then the first open question might be, for example, "How would you like to use this time?" or "How could we use this time to your advantage?"

Usually, the first person to start talking will say something important. Team members should also encourage others to say what was on their minds when they entered the conversation. The purpose of this question is to make room for everyone to participate actively in the discussion and thus reduce the tension they experience. In a serious crisis, participants may be very frightened about a family member's problem or about being blamed for their children's problems, for example. Such fear and tension discourage free discussion. By saying something themselves at the beginning of the discussion, their tension is relieved, and they are more open to listening to what others have to say and expressing their own opinions.

The aim is to create a space for all voices to be heard. Throughout the discussion, members of the treatment team can comment on ideas that come to mind about the nature of the problem and possible treatment methods. It is important that they speak about the participants in the discussion in a respectful way and avoid categorizing the problem with fixed attributes. It is useful to present their own views in the form of reflections, such as "From what Dad said, it occurred to me that this situation might be very difficult for Maja too." Such reflective comments make space and invite others' responses and comments. Moreover, when I speak in the 'I' form, I emphasize throughout that we participate in the dialogue as human beings. I do not seek to express the best interpretation of an issue, but my own view, while waiting for the comments of other speakers.

At the end of the therapy meeting, it is advisable to set aside time for the issues of the clinicians, if they have not already been addressed as part of a naturally flowing dialogue. It is important in this part to raise any suggestions about the treatment plan that seem relevant, such as the choice of appropriate medication and its options. Once this conversation has taken place, it is time to begin to bring the therapy meeting to a close. This is usually a good time to reiterate what has been agreed upon and what has been left unresolved. Personally, I also usually give positive feedback to the participants in the discussion. I might say, "I feel that we have been able to discuss important issues. It seems that we have not been able to resolve all the issues, and it would be good to continue the discussions. Now it's time to call it a day. But before we finish, is there anything else that needs to be added?" In this way, the last word in the discussion is left to the clients. The first words are our clients' words, and the last words are our clients' words. In this way, the experience of being able to influence the course of treatment and of being heard can be conveyed.

All care plans and decisions are also made in the presence of everyone. The pioneer of need-adapted care, Yrjö Alanen (1993), saw the therapy meeting as having three functions: (1) to gather information about the problem, (2) to build a treatment plan and make all necessary decisions based on the diagnosis made in the discussion, and (3) to establish a psychotherapeutic dialogue. The overall focus is on strengthening the adult side of the patient and normalizing the situation, rather than focusing on the pathological side of the behavior. The starting point for treatment is how each family and each family member has, in their own language, named the patient's problem. The treatment team adapts its own way of speaking to each case according to the needs of each one. Problems are seen as socially constructed so that they are reformulated in each conversation (Bakhtin, 1984; Gergen, 2009; Shotter, 1993). Each person present speaks in their own voice, and listening attentively to others and responding to their expressions becomes more important than the interview style. All expressions are accepted, which can be challenging. For example, in a psychotic crisis, it is important to accept the psychotic delusions or hallucinations of the person in need as one voice among others.

Open Dialogue without preconceived themes or forms seems to be important in building a new language for talking about challenging issues. These issues can take many forms, they could have happened at any time, and in fact, any topic of conversation can open the way to a new narrative. Whatever their background, it is important to take the patient's hallucinations, for example, seriously and not to challenge their reality in a crisis situation, especially in the early stages of treatment. Instead, the therapist might ask: "Wait a minute, did I hear you say that you control your neighbor's thoughts? Could you tell me more about how it is possible that you can control other people's thoughts? I haven't been able to do that myself." Others could then be asked, "What do you think about this? How do you understand what M is saying?" The purpose of such a question is to allow a range of voices to be heard on the topics under discussion, including the psychotic experience. If the team can create a reflective atmosphere that allows different and conflicting voices to be heard, the network has the opportunity to build narratives of coping (Stern et al., 1999; Trimble, 2000). This can be one part of a process in which the person of concern and their social network can begin to construct new words for their problems. People often say something unexpected or surprising at the very moment when the most sensitive and crucial issues are being discussed, which may be connected to the still unspoken voices in the body's memory. For example, one might ask: "What did I say wrong when you started talking about it?" or "Wait a minute, what were we talking about when M started talking about how voices control her?" The role of the care team is to allow the patient's network to take the lead in generating content and respond to each statement in a dialogical way to help build new understanding among participants.

One way of responding is to have a discussion among the team members. One part of this discussion is what Andersen called a reflective conversation. In Open Dialogue, no specific reflective team is formed, but members of the team move flexibly from asking questions to discussing with other team members. Sometimes this may require asking permission: "Could you wait a moment so we can discuss what we have started to think about? You can listen; afterward, we will ask for comments on what we have said." Usually, the family and the rest of the social network listen carefully to what the professionals say about their problems. The discussion between the team members has a special role to play because it is in these discussions that treatment plans are built. Everything is transparent. Decisions about hospitalization, the start of possible medication, and the planning of individual psychotherapy are some examples of the content of the discussions and decisions. In each case, the aim is to consider different options, from which a course of action is then chosen. For example, if the situation is so serious that the team is considering the possibility of compulsory treatment, it seems important for staff to be able to discuss openly the need for a compulsory treatment decision and to express their different opinions. Any traditional method of treatment can be used according to the unique needs of the person in the center of concern. He/she may have individual psychotherapy or other therapies (e.g., art therapy, group therapy, and occupational therapy), and the family may meet in family therapy.

The dialogue of an open meeting is a discussion with the family in multi-relational meetings. It may have some of the same features as, say, systemic family therapy, but there are also important differences. Open Dialogue therapy meetings do not focus on exploring the family system and identifying problems or even on communication within the family system. In contrast to traditional systemic family therapy, the aim of dialogue is not to "provide the impetus to change the rigid logic of the system by introducing a new logic" (Boscolo & Bertrando, 1993, p. 217), but to create a shared space for a new language in which issues can begin to take on new meaning. The important thing is to follow the expressions of the clients, accepting them without changing them, so that attention is focused on what they say and not on what their meaning is. In interviews and discussions in systemic family therapy, the therapist often seeks to uncover the behavioral and communicative patterns behind the visible behavior. Open Dialogue discussions focus on building new words and new language by accepting the other person's expression unconditionally. Thus, in a conversation, I may often repeat word for word what the other person said and then encourage them to say more, as, for example "You said it was sad when Dad moved away from home. Would you tell me more about that?"

Open Dialogue is also slightly different from narrative therapy (White & Epston, 1990). Open Dialogue and narrative therapies share a similar understanding of the reality that emerges from people's stories. The narrative therapist encourages all participants to share their views on the same issue in order to create the richest possible collection of descriptions. The aim is to move from thin, problem-filled narratives to thicker stories that begin to have multiple nuances. The therapist can then use his or her own comments to guide the search for unique anomalies in the problem-saturated narratives. The narrative therapist can also focus on finding a word or description that externalizes the problem to help new stories emerge. In narrative therapy, the story has a narrator; in dialogical therapy, a new story is created among the participants. Where the narrative therapist is the active facilitator of the conversation, the dialogical therapist unconditionally follows the words and expressions of clients and follows what happens when we respond to them. What becomes most important is what happens in the here-and-now of our conversation. This is more important than what is being discussed, because really, whatever the topic of discussion, a dialogical shared experience can be built from the discussion.

How to Organize Open Dialogues in an Optimal Way?

Above I have described the process of a therapy meeting and a dialogical therapy conversation involving a team and the person at the center of the concern, alone or with their family and network. Open Dialogue originally evolved as a description of an entire psychiatric treatment system. The development in this direction in the Tornio region began in 1984 when we started to organize therapy meetings at Keropudas Hospital. Through various stages, the whole psychiatric system was transformed into an integrated community care system so that mobile crisis teams started to make home visits in the most severe crises throughout the hospital district. After this model had been in operation for about 5 years, we studied the optimal factors for a good outcome of the new model of care under the guidance of Professor Jukka Aaltonen (Aaltonen et al., 2011).

We analyzed the course of treatment of all patients who were first admitted to the hospital over a 10-year period (1985–1994) and selected patients who were for the first time admitted for psychotic problems. By comparing hospital-centered care with this new, predominantly home-based or otherwise outpatient crisis response, we found the key principles of the new approach. The big difference between the two periods was that in the 1980s, psychosis was treated in hospitals, whereas after the establishment of the new crisis clinic in Tornio and Kemi, psychotic problems were treated mainly at home.

The best treatment process seemed to take place in the following situation:

1. Treatment starts by organizing the first therapy meeting immediately on the first day of contact.
2. The patient's social network is involved both at the beginning and during treatment. The most important part of the social network is, of course, the patient's family, but it is also important to take into account other networks, such as friends, classmates in a crisis at school, or neighbors.
3. Flexible care that takes into account the unique needs of each patient and family and selects the most appropriate methods for those who need help. One manifestation of flexibility is that the care team moves to the patient's home or other locations according to the needs of the family. For example, in the case of medication, each patient's unique needs are always assessed. In the most severe cri-

ses, such as psychotic problems, neuroleptic medication is not started immediately, but only after it may have been established that the other active psychosocial measures chosen are not sufficient. Any psychotherapeutic or other methods may be used as part of the overall treatment.
4. The care team takes responsibility for the organization of care and all care decisions, which are made in joint therapy meetings. The care system takes responsibility for all contacts. The staff member who takes the request for help is responsible for organizing the first joint therapy meeting, which then decides who are the best members of the "case-specific team" that takes responsibility for the treatment process. Staff members are not allowed to say, "This is not our problem; please contact the A-Clinic" (for example), but the clinician should confirm that they will arrange a meeting and invite the A-Clinic therapist to attend if they suspect that alcohol or drug overuse is contributing to the problem.
5. Building psychological continuity of care across the boundaries of the different providers so that the case-specific team can include, for example, a social worker together with a mental health nurse. Similarly, the same team can include both psychiatric outpatients and hospital staff.
6. Treatment is structured as a process that tolerates uncertainty and hears the voices of all family members and other participants in therapy meetings equally.
7. The primary focus of treatment is on creating a shared understanding of the family's life and what is involved in the crisis. To this end, the focus is on creating a dialogue rather than on eliminating the patient's symptoms or changing the family.

In doing the research, we immediately realized that these conclusions in fact describe a new approach to care, building on the tradition of the need-adapted approach originally developed in Turku (Alanen, 1993). We first publicly referred to this system of care as Open Dialogue in 1995 (Seikkula et al., 1995). The name Open Dialogue emerged as a conclusion of the research findings. Without research, the whole system of Open Dialogue would not exist as we recognize it today. This observation is very important for the message of my book: Dialogical practices cannot be transferred from one place to another by adopting principles established elsewhere and then faithfully following them. Following principles taken from outside is not dialogical practice, because the basic event of dialogicity is responding to the other in the here and now on the terms of the situation. Thus, what are called the principles of Open Dialogue must also be understood as the crystallization of the research into the optimally implemented treatment process. Knowledge of these results can then help each individual to improve his or her own performance within his or her team.

The Dialogical Care Experience Has a Lifelong Impact

Optimal implementation of the principles of Open Dialogue seems to create the best conditions for mobilizing the resources of the person at the center of concern, his/her family, and social network in a crisis. Several studies have demonstrated the effectiveness of the Open Dialogue approach implemented in Western Lapland compared to conventional treatment. I will review some of these studies later in Chap. 9 when I discuss the importance of scientific research in developing a dialogical approach.

Here I briefly describe just one study to illustrate how radical the change is. When followed the treatment of patients who contacted because of the first psychotic crisis, it was found astonishingly large differences compared to Treatment-as-Usual Finnish psychiatric care, on average 19 years after the start of treatment (Bergström et al., 2018) (Table 1.1).

Open Dialogue therapy seems to create a completely different way of coping with difficult crises. In conventional treatment, patients were hospitalized for more than a month in almost all cases; they used neuroleptic medication much more at the beginning of treatment than at follow-up; half of patients in conventional treatment were still in contact with treatment compared to less than a third of those in Open Dialogue treatment. The most dramatic difference is that two out of three patients in conventional treatment are on disability pension compared to one-third of those who had Open Dialogue treatment 19 years earlier.

Table 1.1 Use of psychiatric care and disability pensions 19 years after the first psychotic crisis (%)

	Western Cape Open Dialogue ($N = 108$)	The treatment—as usual rest of Finland ($N = 1763$)	p
More than 30 days of hospitalization	18.5	94	***[a]
Neuroleptics at the start of treatment	16.7	75.5	***
Neuroleptics at the time of monitoring	36.1	81.1	***
Treatment contact continues	27.8	49.2	***
On invalidity pension	33	61	***

[a] In the tables in the book, *** indicates the strongest statistical significance ($p < 0.001$), ** indicates a significant statistical difference ($p < 0.010$) and * indicates a statistical significance at the level of a suggestive of an effect $p < 0.05$

The Importance of Drugs Is Declining

One factor contributing to this exceptionally promising result is the fact that Open Dialogue has made it possible to substantially reduce the use of neuroleptics in the treatment of psychosis. Neuroleptic drugs for psychosis have many side effects, which can be prevented by creating an encounter that mobilizes the person's own resources in Open Dialogue. Neuroleptic medication can cause tardive dyskinesia, obesity, and a general flattening of emotional life. All these factors can play a decisive role in the loss of an active attitude to life. In addition to these, there is a large body of research evidence in recent years that neuroleptic medication is associated with more rapid destruction of brain tissue in schizophrenia patients (Ho et al., 2011), increased mortality (Joukamaa et al., 2006), disability, and prolonged need for treatment (Bergström et al., 2020).

In the Open Dialogue in Acute Psychosis study, only about 25% of patients with first-time psychosis were taking neuroleptic medication during the first 2 years of the study. This first 2-year treatment experience seems to have a lifelong impact, so that in the event of a re-emergence crisis, not nearly as much neuroleptic medication needs to be prescribed, even if they are no longer in the Open Dialogue service, but in conventional psychiatric care. Indeed, the positive experience of the first treatment seems to have increased the patients' resources, reducing the need for neuroleptics and protecting them from adverse effects.

As far as conventional psychiatric care is concerned, attention is drawn to the worrying fact that the outcomes for psychotic patients are very similar to those of the 1980s. In conventional care, there seems to have been no improvement in the treatment of psychotic problems over the last 30 years. It is indeed high time to start developing a humane approach.

What to Improve in Dialogue: Suggested Answers and Book Chapters

Dialogue is about helping people in a humane way. It is reasonable to ask what makes dialogical care better and what makes it such a much more effective way of dealing with difficult crises. As these results have so far only been obtained from studies in Western Lapland, it is also important to consider what the most important factors are when working in a dialogical way so that they can be applied elsewhere and also outside psychiatry.

Open Dialogue in Western Lapland is based on a long-standing tradition of development and research and the training of staff. The results are not based on a simple new method, but on a profound change in the way of thinking and caring. The curative power of the dialogical approach seems to be based on the following factors:

1. Dialogical practice creates a new view of the human, in which the best mental health treatment is acceptance of one's emotional experiences rather than eliminating psychological symptoms or aiming at changing families (Chap. 3).
2. Dialogical practice adopts and makes use of the latest intersubjective knowledge that human beings are active participants in interaction rhythmically and bodily from birth. Reality is always created in relation. The treatment of severe mental health crises considers the person as a full human being, embodied participant in a constantly evolving stream of interaction, in dialogue (Chap. 4).
3. Open Dialogue has evolved as family therapy work so that the aim is no longer to change the family system but to create a shared experience in which a new language for managing the most difficult experiences emerges. Families are not the objects of treatment but indispensable partners to the team (Chap. 5).
4. Dialogical practice draws on the knowledge that the human mind is constructed as a bodily process that allows the human being to be considered as a whole, thus transcending the dualistic concept of the human being. Reality is contextual, arising in each situation. The embodied understanding of the human mind makes psychotherapy possible to a much greater extent than before because there is no longer a special inner linguistic insight needed, but the very act of sharing a feeling is healing (Chap. 6).
5. Dialogical practice makes it possible to understand psychotic behavior as a necessary response to extreme stress. Psychosis is not a psychopathological condition or illness, and people have many resources of their own to cope with a crisis. This has made it possible to significantly reduce the use of neuroleptic medication and prevent its side effects (Chap. 7).
6. The dialogical orientation has created ways of determining the quality of the dialogue. Improving dialogues can be explored to find the best ways to help others and thus develop a conversation that supports clients' own reflection (Chap. 8).
7. Open Dialogue is based on systematic scientific research conducted in practical treatment situations in naturalistic research settings. The role of scientific research is to develop the practice in a broad sense, exploring both treatment outcomes and dialogical processes, as has happened in Open Dialogue. I know of no other psychiatric treatment model that has been scientifically studied so extensively (Chap. 9).

These are my suggestions in response to the healing power of dialogue. The book is structured so that I deal with each topic in its own chapter to build an overall response. In the next chapter, I will describe one Open Dialogue meeting with the aim of gaining an even more detailed image of the challenges and opportunities created by dialogical encounters.

References

Aaltonen, J., Seikkula, J., & Lehtinen, K. (2011). Comprehensive open-dialogue approach I: Developing a comprehensive culture of need-adapted approach in a psychiatric public health catchment area the Western Lapland Project. *Psychosis, 3*, 179–191.

Alanen, Y. (1993). *Schizophrenia. Causes and appropriate treatment*. Routledge.

Andersen, T. (1991). *The reflecting team*. Norton.

Andersen, T. (1995). Reflecting processes; Acts of forming and informing. In S. Friedman (Ed.), *The reflecting team in action* (pp. 11–37). Guilford.

Andersen, T. (2022). *Wandering and turning points. A book about touch, involvement in psychiatry and other peace work*.

Anderson, H. (1997). *Conversation, language, and possibilities: A postmodern approach to therapy*. Basic Books.

Anderson, H., & Goolishian, H. (1988). Human systems as linguistic systems: Preliminary and evolving ideas about the implications for clinical theory. *Family Process, 27*, 371–393.

Bakhtin, M. (1984). *Problems of Dostoyevsky's poetics: Theory and history of literature* (Vol. 8). Manchester University Press.

Bakhtin, M. (1986). *Speech genres and other late essays*. University of Texas Press.

Baxter, L. A. (2004). Dialogues of relating. In R. Anderson, L. A. Baxter, & K. N. Cissna (Eds.), *Dialogues: Theorizing difference in communication studies* (pp. 107–124). Sage.

Bergström, T., Seikkula, J., Alakare, B., Mäki, P., Köngäs-Saviaro, P., Taskila, J. J., et al. (2018). The family-oriented Open Dialogue approach in the treatment of first-episode psychosis: Nineteen-year outcomes. *Psychiatry Research, 270*, 168–175.

Bergström, T., Taskila, J., Alakare, B., Köngäs-Saviaro, P., Miettunen, J., & Seikkula, J. (2020). Five-year cumulative exposure to antipsychotic medication after first-episode psychosis and its association with 19-year outcomes. *Schizophrenia Bulletin Open*. https://doi.org/10.1093/schizbullopen/sgaa050

Boscolo, L., & Bertrando, P. (1993). *The times of time*. Norton.

Furman, B., & Ahola, T. (2020). *From problems to solutions. Fundamentals of brief therapy*.

Gergen, K. (2009). *Relational being: Beyond self and community*. Oxford University Press.

Haarakangas, K. (1997). *Voices of the treatment meeting*. Jyväskylä Studies in Education, Psychology and Social Research, 130.

Hermans, H. J. M. (2004). The dialogical self: Between exchange and power. In H. J. M. Hermans & G. Dimaggio (Eds.), *The dialogical self in psychotherapy* (pp. 13–28). Brunner/Routledge.

Ho, B.-C., Andreasen, N., Ziebell, S., Pierson, R., & Magnotta, V. (2011). Long-term antipsychotic treatment and brain volumes a longitudinal study of first-episode schizophrenia. *Archives of General Psychiatry, 68*(2), 128–137.

Joukamaa, M., Heliovaara, M., Knekt, P., Aromaa, A., Raitasalo, R., & Lehtinen, V. (2006). Schizophrenia, neuroleptic medication and mortality. *The British Journal of Psychiatry, 188*, 122–127.

Kim Berg, I. (2001). *Tales of solutions*. Norton.

Leiman, M. (2004). Dialogical sequence analysis. In H. Hermans & C. Dimaggio (Eds.), *The dialogical self in psychotherapy* (pp. 255–270). Brunner-Routledge.

Levinas, I. (1985). *Ethics and infinity*. Duquesne University Press.

Lysaker, P., & Lysaker, J. (2004). Dialogical transformation in the psychotherapy of schizophrenia. In H. Hermans & C. Dimaggio (Eds.), *The dialogical self in psychotherapy* (pp. 205–219). Brunner/Routledge.

Olson, M., Seikkula, J., & Ziedonis, D. (2014). *The key elements of dialogic practice in Open Dialogue*. The University of Massachusetts Medical School.

Rober, P. (2017). *In therapy together. Family therapy as dialogue*. Palgrave.

Seikkula, J., Aaltonen, J., Alakare, B., Haarakangas, K., Sutela, M., & Keränen, J. (1995). Treating psychosis by means of Open Dialogue. In S. Friedman (Ed.), *The reflecting team in action: Collaborative practice in family therapy*. Guilford Press.

Seikkula, J., & Arnkil, T. E. (2014). *Open dialogues and anticipations. Respecting otherness in the present moment*. TH.
Sempere, J., & Fuenzalida, C. (2017). *Terapias multifamiliares: El modelo interfamiliar: la terapia hecha entre todos*. Psimatica.
Shotter, J. (1993). *Cultural politics of every day life. Social constructionism, rhetoric and knowing of the third kind*. Open University Press.
Steiner, G. (1989). *Real presences: Is there anything in what we say*. University of Chicago Press.
Stern, D. (2004). *The present moment in psychotherapy and everyday life*. Norton.
Stern, S., Doolan, M., Stables, E., Szmukler, G., & Eisler, I. (1999). Disruption and reconstruction: Narrative insights into the experience of family members caring for a relative diagnosed with serious mental illness. *Family Process, 38*(3), 353–369.
Stiles, B., Osatuke, K., Click, M., & MacKay, H. (2004). Encounters between internal voices generate emotion: An elaboration of the assimilation model. In H. Hermans & C. Dimaggio (Eds.), *The dialogical self in psychotherapy* (pp. 91–107). Brunner/Routledge.
Trimble, D. (2000). Emotion and voice in network therapy. *Netletter, 7*(1), 11–16.
Wertsch, J. V. (1991). *Voices of the mind: A sociocultural approach to mediated action*. Harvard University Press.
White, M., & Epston, D. (1990). *Narrative means to therapeutic ends*. Norton.

Chapter 2 "I've Never Seen Anything Like This Before"

I would like to continue the introduction to the topic of this book with two examples of the surprising power of dialogical practice. The first example comes from the first experience of Open Dialogue in Barcelona and the second from a family consultation in a major South American city, where I, myself, was a facilitator. This is an example of an Open Dialogue meeting. There has been much international interest in the development and research into dialogical practice. At the time of writing this book, for example, Open Dialogue training programs have been or are being implemented in about 40 countries. A seminar was held in the city in question, during which we also met the family and the team.

One of the basic ideas behind the practice of Open Dialogue is that clinicians form a team to work together with those who need help. The team members do not plan a therapy meeting in advance, but all discussions are, in reality, open. Another basic idea is that any discussion about understanding the problem is open so that the people in need help are involved from the very beginning in the conversation. The open discussion of all the important issues creates a very productive tension in which the people who need help become the authors of their own life stories in a situation that may seem desperate.

The Power of Dialogue Can Surprise

The first experiences of dialogical practice may surprise you with their intensity. Jordi, a Spanish psychiatrist, sent me an email about his own experiences. Jordi has over 40 years of experience in psychiatry, is also a trained psychoanalyst and has a lot of experience in psychotherapy. With his permission, I am publishing part of his letter, as it illustrates well the surprising nature of dialogical practice.

> Dear Jaakko. We met in Madrid at the Open Dialogue seminar. At dinner we discussed the possibility of applying Open Dialogue in my mental health center. I felt that you encouraged me to give it a try.

J. Seikkula, *Why Dialogue Does Cure*,
https://doi.org/10.1007/978-3-031-91294-8_2

> Well, we did. We started with the first cases right after the seminar. One case was a young woman who had her first psychotic experience. The team was: a social worker, a male nurse and myself. In some of the discussions also a psychologist. We have had 20 sessions with the patient, her family and her network. The result is absolutely shocking. We stopped the medication after four months (20 mg olanzapine). She found a new job after three months, got her driver's license and recently started university studies.
>
> We have now worked with the Open Dialogue style in eight cases. The different teams include two social workers, two nurses, two psychiatrists and a psychologist. We have a senior psychologist, a family therapist as a supervisor.
>
> I am writing this letter if you or your team would like to share our experiences, or perhaps there is a network of teams working in the same way. How can we learn more about your system?
>
> Best regards Jordi.

Jordi's letter was surprising to me in many ways. Over the years, I have come to think that dialogical practice is very challenging to adopt and that even the basics require training. This is an assumption I have made after seeing many attempts and failures. We may set far too high goals for ourselves. It can also be difficult to adopt a dialogical approach because in our training, we are used to learning how to manage different problems, understand their causes and develop specific therapeutic interventions to manage or eliminate this or that symptom. Dialogical meetings are about meeting the person, not treating the symptom. Moreover, psychiatric practice reinforces the focus on symptom by emphasizing in the treatment of excellence guidelines the specific treatment method for each illness and each symptom. The whole chain of reasoning in psychiatric care is based on symptom-centeredness. Unfortunately, this logic is also taking hold in the field of psychotherapy, with some therapeutic approaches designing their own therapeutic methods for different symptoms. Often, therapists' habitual ways of working seem to raise the bar for dialogicity, because in difficult situations, we easily suppose that we need specific interventions to manage the situations. But Jordi wrote that after one seminar and a subsequent discussion at the dinner table, they decided as a team to make a change. And they did. They started with some selected people with psychotic problems. From his description, I saw that they had managed to adopt the key elements of the practice of open dialogue from the very beginning. They modified their work to work as a team with clients, they were open to inviting family and also the wider social network to join in, and they also encouraged the individual therapist to participate in joint dialogues from time to time.

"The Result Is Shocking"

And then Jordi wrote: "*The result is absolutely shocking*." After such a long working experience, you would think that Jordi would have experienced everything. But the dialogical approach gave him and his team a real surprise. Their patient returned to her studies and work, acquired new skills, and stopped taking neuroleptic medication. These events go against the basic assumptions of mainstream psychiatry. Psychotic problems are said to be primarily brain-based problems for which the basic treatment is usually very long-term or end-of-life psychotropic medication. Only about a third are expected to recover and return to a full, social life. But in dialogical practice, it is possible to achieve quite a different result, as this working group found in individual cases and as we have observed in systematic follow-up studies in Western Lapland. After 2 years, even more than 90% of those who have recovered from a psychotic crisis for the first time have been able to return to work (Seikkula et al., 2011). The impact of this experience was so great that even after 19 years, the difference with conventional treatment was still shocking, as we noted earlier.

Sharing Family Grief

Another example is a family consultation that revealed great grief of one family and the importance of sharing it. The dialogical approach is very different from traditional psychiatric care, where the staff usually plan the care among themselves. Thus, a male psychiatrist in his 50 s who was participating in the seminar and followed the consultation, said that he had never seen anything like this in his entire career. He also stated dramatically that he felt as if his brain was about to explode. He went on to say that he needs to completely reevaluate his own practice with his own patients.

Based on the conversation, I think he was particularly impressed by the personal nature of the discussion, in which the clinicians were also moved and were ready to share their own experiences. They also showed their own emotions openly. I was also moved as I listened to the stories of the family and the therapists. This is a very different approach from the systemic family therapy training I received in the 1980s. That training emphasized the need for the family therapist to be neutral and not to show their own feelings. The family therapist was also instructed to use a special frame interview, which focused on to talk about the actions and behavior of the family members, not their feelings. Now, in dialogical work, I actually do the opposite. I want to make space for the emotional experience of the problem. When the emotional experiences come out, the therapist becomes part of this emotional world. As mentioned in the previous chapter, we always participate in the dialogue with our own personal voices, according to our own life experiences. Therapists participate in dialogue in a much more personal way than in the early 1980s family therapy guidelines. All deep dialogues are also experienced in our bodies. My bodily sensation becomes part of the shared encounter because it is always a response to something that is happening in that particular interaction.

The family we met in the consultation[1] had three generations, the mother, her two daughters and the 13-year-old son of one daughter. Not much was said about the daughters' father, but we learned that the parents had divorced when the girls were very young, and the father was occasionally involved in their lives. The family problem was dealt with by a team consisting mainly of three members, Alfonso, the psychiatrist; Leticia, the psychologist; and Rocio the nurse. Other services were often needed because of the very difficult situation of the family. This is also part of the daily routine of Open Dialogue care. It involves all the professionals involved in a person or family problem, according to the needs of each case. In dialogue work, we always involve the family's own social network.

Helena, the mother, and her daughter Natalia were present for the discussion. Another older daughter, Liisa, followed the dialogue via video with her son Cristof. Liisa had stayed at home because travelling with Cristof was challenging. Cristof had lost his mobility and speech and needed round-the-clock support due to an illness that had been going on for 10 years and had gradually progressed. As the conversation later revealed, this was an insurmountable burden for his mother.

Opening the Conversation: What Do Team Members Expect?

A space at the front of the seminar room was reserved for the discussion. Leticia welcomed everyone and gave the floor to me. I spent the first 9 min talking with the team members. I asked them what made them invite the family to this discussion and what their expectations were. Leticia said she wanted to have space for her own thoughts because working with the family had been very challenging. Alfonso said he wanted to get clarity on his uncertainty about not having done enough to help the family. Finally, Rocio said he wanted to reflect in particular on Liisa's situation. She said that she was particularly affected by the difficult situation of Liisa in the family. Everyone nodded and said that Rocio was a very special support person for her. I also asked them what they expected from me. Did they want to faclitate the conversation and for me to listen and comment on their conversation? Or do they want me to be an active interviewer? All three of them said that they wanted me to lead the discussion, which naturally suited me, because it was important for me to do exactly what they wanted.

This part of the conversation is familiar to Open Dialogue. In general, in care situations where there is no external consultant, all discussions take place in the open, in the presence of those who need help. This includes those conversations in which clinicians talk openly about their own observations and ideas that guide their care. In Open Dialogues, there is often no clear division of labor as to who leads the discussion and who listens. But in this kind of consultation, it is important because

[1] I have changed the main points of the case and the names of the participants to protect their privacy. This also applies to all other descriptions of therapeutic dialogues in this book.

I was a consultant in their therapeutic process. So, it is very important to define my role in the conversation, which is likely to be the only meeting for me with this family and the caring team. This kind of work is also a very good orientation for live supervision, where those who need help are present, both the family and the team.

As we were not in a hurry, the discussion was calm and reflective. As part of the discussion, Leticia told us that they had started working with the family 3 years earlier, when Natalia had been hospitalized for psychotic problems. This had been repeated three times, but now Natalia's life was going well. She had completed her university studies and was working as a teacher. A year earlier, Helena, the mother of the family, had contacted her because Liisa had made a serious suicide attempt. Since then, Liisa had made several suicide attempts and talked all day about not wanting to live because life was so difficult because of caring for Cristof. It was because of this challenging problem that the team wanted this consultation with the family.

After my discussion with the therapists, I turned to Helena and Natalia to ask how they wanted to use this time. Again, this is a very typical opening to an Open Dialogue. We, therapists, do not direct the discussion to certain topics, but the absolute guideline is to follow the topics that need to be raised by the person who needs help. This opened the next few minutes of discussion.

"I Have Failed as a Mother"

Jaakko Well, I'm very curious to hear what it was like for you to come here today and what specific expectations you have for our discussion[2]?

Helena Good morning. I'm Helena. I am the mother of Natalia and Liisa. Yes, I've always wanted an answer to why both of my daughters have the same problem. Both of them have been in hospital, one of them, Liisa, because of depression, because she lost the will to live. Natalia had a psychotic episode and lost the plot in her life. For me as a mother, as a mother of two daughters, it is very difficult… I have no answers to what happened.

Jaakko Yes, I hear you saying that you want to get an answer to what happened when your daughter had similar problems?

Helena Yes, because as a mother, you ask what I did wrong. Even though you were doing your best, you failed. Do you understand? Liisa didn't want to… she lost the will to live because she has a little boy who was a normal child until he was three and a half, so to speak. Now he is a 13-year-old special child. He doesn't walk, he doesn't talk, he can't hear. He is totally dependent on his mother. Liisa gave up her own life to live her child's life today. As for Natalia, I don't know what happened.

[2] This conversation was interpreted simultaneously into everyone's earbuds. I spoke English and the others spoke their native language. This meant that I was not always quite sure of their choice of words and expressions.

Now she has succeeded in her life and her profession. Sometimes, I ask myself what I did wrong.
Jaakko Yes, I heard you say that you think to yourself what you did wrong. How did you fail?
Helena Yes, because as a mother I feel like a failure. Why did this happen to my daughters? (Moves and tears fall)

(8).[3]

"I Feel Sadness in My Stomach"

Jaakko I hear you say that as a mother I failed…
Helena Yes, for me…
Jaakko When I hear what you say, I get a little sad. When I feel sad, I often feel it here (strokes his upper stomach with his hand). Now I feel a little sad.
Helena That's how I feel.
Jaakko Yes. Thank you for saying that. (5) Natalia? What was it like for you to come here today, and what expectations do you have for us today?
Natalia I like this style of therapy that is offered to us, it seems very reasonable. I have talked more with Liisa than with my mother in the past because my mother has not been able to attend our meetings lately. I like this because we can talk about anything. We each talk a bit, they (the therapists) come in and ask more questions. It feels really good to me. But today, what makes me feel uncomfortable, as Rocio said, is that my sister doesn't seem to feel the same way.

So, I ask myself, what is my role? Am I trying to talk and bring her in, really get her involved so that she understands that this is not just for me. No one has ever said that this therapy is just for Natalia. I had problems, and I needed therapy. But they didn't say at the time that Natalia needed therapy. It's for the whole family! I feel uncomfortable because my sister doesn't see the same way, that this will benefit her. Mum is supersensitive about this. She has talked and helped without grumbling. But for my sister, it doesn't make sense. So, that is what I'm looking forward to from this discussion today is: What is my role with my sister? To give her the freedom to decide how to engage in our conversations and how she might make sense of these conversations.

The conversation with Helena and Natalia seemed very easy. They both immediately started to talk openly about their concerns. Several very important things

[3] The numbers in brackets in the discussions refer to the length of the pause in the speech. If there are only brackets, the pause was very short.

happened in terms of the dialogue. First of all, and perhaps most importantly, an absolute effort was made to get to the bottom of their experiences. That is why I repeated the words they used at several points. This is important for two reasons. It is a way of ensuring that we are really following their experience and not adding our own interpretation to it. If we repeat an essential part of their experience, those who need help may also hear something about their own experience that they have not heard before. So, when they say something, they may be saying it for the first time, and if someone else repeats what they say word for word, they may hear what they said to themselves. Secondly, in this way, we keep in check the impulses in our own minds to make interpretations and give meanings according to our therapeutic orientation. The basic premise of a dialogical discussion is that we are able to reflect and reassess our own feelings and thoughts all the time and give space to the words and related experiences of those who need help. When this becomes possible, those who need help can find new resources to live with their own difficult situation. Again, the important thing is to express the experience and hear it for themselves, not to give their experience a particular meaning, for example, by interpreting what they say in some way. Some other therapeutic approaches talk about the importance of the therapist repeating the client's message in other words. For me, it is important for dialogicity to repeat their message exactly in their words.

What bothered me a little in this conversation was that I couldn't quite accurately repeat what they said because our conversation was interpreted into English through earphones and so I could never be quite sure that what was translated for me was accurately told in the words they used. I felt, however, that I was gradually able to pick up something essential from what the mother was saying, because already in the second turn of speech she herself was in tears, saying that as a mother she had failed and would like to discuss it. Could there be a more relevant subject for discussion? My experience is that, in general, open questions at the beginning of a discussion are answered by those who need help with something that seems very relevant. I don't have to worry about whether this is the most important topic of discussion because a dialogical and healing experience can arise from discussing a wide range of topics.

Right at the beginning of Helena's speech, I felt a very strong feeling in my stomach. I also put this into words by saying that I felt sadness, which often feels like pressure in the diaphragm area. One participates in the dialogue with one's whole body. Recently, I have become more interested in how this happens and in how it relates to the dialogue spoken with words. We'll come back to this later (Chap. 6). To this Helena responded by confirming that this is how she feels. There were also several moments of silence in the conversation, the longest being when Helena said she had failed as a mother. Later in the conversation, it emerged that this was very surprising to both Natalia and the team, who said that the mother had never talked about her feelings before. And now she was forming words for her most distressing experiences while being moved.

"What if They Were Here to Hear?"

Natalia began to talk about her difficult relationship with her sister, who did not trust the conversations but often said that these conversations were for Natalia and not for her. At the same time, Natalia also said that she had found this approach very helpful. We continued to discuss these issues and Natalia's and Helena's experiences. My interest in how Liisa and Cristof experienced these things was growing. They were not able to join the conversation, and I wanted to get their voices more involved in the discussion. At around the 25 min from the start, I invited their voices into the dialogue by asking Natalia and Helena, her mother, to reflect on what they might have said if they were present.

Jaakko I'm curious to know what you think that if Liisa were here today and had heard what we've talked about so far, what she would say now. Natalia?
Natalia I think she would feel uncomfortable because… I don't know how she would feel physically being here, but I think she would feel uncomfortable … correct me if I'm wrong (turns to Helena) … the way we sit here, I think she would feel embarrassed to sit here as the center of everything. And I also think she would feel uncomfortable because she always comes back to the question of "this therapy is not for me, how can I feel more involved in this?" So, she might feel very uncomfortable.
Jaakko And you think that she would also ask herself here, "Why am I not included in this?"
Natalia No, she might not say it out loud. But I got the impression that she would feel that way. "I'm here for Natalia, it doesn't matter to me." Somehow, this is how her discomfort could be.
Jaakko What…what would you say to her? If…she was here and she felt such uncomfortable feelings, what would you say to her?
Natalia What I usually say to her. Yesterday, when she said she wasn't coming here today, I said it again like this. I would answer that I am happy about it, but I don't expect her to just please me, because therapy is not just for me. It's for Mum, it's for her, it's for Cristof, even if he can't talk or listen, it's for the whole family. Today I am asking for help on how to make my sister feel part of this project because I feel so good about it. I don't want this to continue just for me, I want her too. For example, I am super proud of my mom for being able to see that Liisa wants more help because of Cristof. Something I never thought my mom would think because she didn't think so before therapy. I can already see small changes in our family that weren't there before therapy.
Jaakko Now…what you're saying is that you're saying your mother thinks Liisa needs more help to look after Cristof?
Natalia I think that this therapy model proposed to us helps us to see some things, our difficulties. And I used my mother as an example that my mother can now see something that I realized before, but before the therapy she didn't see it. And I think my sister is failing to take full advantage of the therapy. So, my discomfort…it's not really discomfort, it's sadness for her.

(8)

Jaakko What about…Cristof. He's thirteen now? If he still had words, what would he say about our conversation now?
Helena That he loves us. He would say that he loves us. Because with his gestures, he's always telling us that he loves us. And those were his last words (moves violently, starts crying). "Grandma. I love you with all the love in the universe!" These words were left because he never spoke again after that. He used to say it to us every day. "Mummy, I love you with the universe," "Auntie, I love you with the universe," "Grandma, I love you with the universe." And he said it every day. In his own way, hugging, kissing, he says he loves us beyond measure. And I do everything I can to see my daughters and grandchildren happy. That is my life's purpose.

In working with Open Dialogue, I am used to thinking that we are trying to have a multi-voiced discussion, where there are many different voices present all the time, and not just one correct view. These multiple voices are on two levels, horizontal and vertical, as my colleague Kauko Haarakangas explained in his doctoral thesis. In this conversation, the horizontal voices are heard through the words and other communications of those present, but the internal vertical voices in their experiences are only heard if we invite them into the dialogue. A familiar way for me is to say "If Alice were here and heard this conversation, what would she say?" This seems a bit of a complicated formulation, but it is actually very important. We want the voices of different people and different experiences to be part of the dialogue, not just our assumed opinions. Dialogue always happens here and now. In the dialogue we had, first, Natalia started talking about her sister and the kind of conversation they had in the past. According to her, this would be repeated in our dialogue as well. According to Natalia, the central problem is that Liisa keeps saying that the meetings are helpful for Natalia and for her mother but that they are not helpful for Liisa herself. She said she was sad that Liisa does not benefit from the therapy meetings.

The atmosphere became even sadder when I asked what Cristof would have said if he still had words. Helena replied that he said he loved them. As she said this, she began to cry and told that his last words were that he loved everyone in the amount of a universe. We were all deeply moved. Perhaps the last words this little man ever said were that he loved his family beyond measure.

"I Was Deeply Moved when I Heard Cristof's Voice"

After this part of the discussion, I also wanted to hear more about the experiences of the team members, both from this discussion and from their experiences in general. After about half an hour of discussion, I turn to them.

Jaakko I would like to hear your thoughts. How has our discussion been so far?
Rocio I was deeply moved when I heard Cristof's voice, as Helena said.

Leticia Me too…and I remember in our first conversation, we were waiting for Natalia to come with her mother…and all four of them did. So, I think Cristof is here with us (voice weakens, starts crying).
Alfonso I was very moved too. It was touching. And I think that we included, in our thinking about how to include Liisa, we ended up paying a little more attention to Cristof.
Jaakko Could you say a little bit more?
Alfonso …I think that we, maybe…I kind of want to hug this family, to take it in my arms and each family member individually. And I find myself thinking about how little I've been able to, metaphorically, take Cristof's attention or acknowledge his potential voice in our conversation. And thinking about that now, I'm starting to feel like I can…breathe a little more freely…air (sighs deeply and smiles).
Jaakko I also have a very strong feeling…and although so far, we have only met Helena and Natalia and not Liisa and Cristof, I have a feeling of a family of four very strong people. Each has their own unique place in the world, in the family, and each has their own concerns and perhaps things they enjoy. It was very moving to hear Cristof's voice about his love for family. Likewise, how Natalia spoke of her sister with great love and care. And at the same time…each one has their own place… how shall I put it…their own autonomy. I don't know if that's the right word, but each one has "my place" and a sense of being one.

(11)

Jaakko Some thoughts about what did your therapists think?
Natalia Well…I'm a super fan of this way of working, so it works for me. If you ask me how to improve it, I think we already have everything! Today, listening to my mom, I felt overwhelmed because my mom is very reserved, she doesn't usually talk about her feelings. And now to see her bring all these things here with great understanding…it makes me feel even more…When I try…if my sister wants to, because therapy doesn't work if the person doesn't want to, she can also bring her own issues as a person, as a mother and everything else. So, I really like this model and how our therapists work. It works for me!
Helena Ahh…for me, each one of them is special. Dr. Alfonso, Leti, Rocio, they help us very, very much. I wish very much that Liisa would let herself be helped because sometimes she becomes so rebellious and doesn't let herself be helped. It worries me very much. She…not that she doesn't like Dr. Alfonso and Leticia, but Rocio is very special to her. She always says, "I want to bring you home with me." But they are all very special and mean a lot to my family. I have come to love them very much.

The team members said they were particularly moved when Helena started talking about what Cristof would have said. When Leticia spoke first, she not only said she was moved, but when she told them how she felt, she started to cry. Rocio, and later Alfonso also said they felt moved, and Rocio, when speaking, also started to cry. As I was talking to them, I too became more and more moved, and it was difficult for me to hold back the tears. It was easy for me to understand their experiences. I particularly liked Alfonso's experience, which he shared when I asked him to tell me more. Now Alfonso said he can breathe better. I was immediately reminded of his wish at the beginning of the conversation, when he had been unsure whether he had helped the family enough. When a therapist can breathe more freely, it often means that they are more open to discovering new perspectives. I also shared my own feelings in the conversation. I wanted to add some personal thoughts that had not yet been said. I felt it was important to emphasize the heavy burden that all four family members carried and how masterfully they had coped. This was my genuine feeling. I never say anything that I do not really think.

This part is very typical of Open Dialogue therapy meetings. Clinicians reflect aloud on their own thoughts and feelings in front of the family. Repeatedly, those who need help say they like this, often even looking forward to this point in the discussion. After this discussion of the team members, it is important to always ask those in need what came to their minds while listening to the therapists. It was very illustrative that Helena started talking about the therapist using affectionate names for them. That illustrates how important therapists had become to the family and at the same time, professionally helped them deeply.

"Suffering Has Every Right to be Bitter"

We continued to discuss their experiences of Liisa's difficult situation. Both family members and therapists participated in this discussion together. I also asked what greetings each of them would like to send to Lisa and Cristof. Mum and Natalia promised to tell them what they had thought during the conversation. Natalia particularly liked one of my comments in which I said that Liisa had every right to feel bitter about her life because she had experienced such unfair things. In fact, each of us thought of good wishes for Lisa. Personally, I suggested that we could somehow convey to Liisa the tears we had shared in the conversation. At the very end, I asked everyone how they had experienced the conversation. At this point, Alfonso said that he had received an accepting hug from me, which gave him strength. Rocio said he liked Alfonso's comment about having more space to breathe. Family members said they had been heard. They also said that they have learned to listen to each other more and more in all conversations. When I asked for their thoughts on what Liisa and Cristof would have said, Helena said that Liisa said "Oh, I wish I had been part of this conversation!"

In total, our conversation lasted 1 h and 8 min. I was very relaxed, even though we had discussed such a difficult family situation. After 2 weeks, the therapists met with the family and watched a video of the meeting. And sure enough, Liisa said, "Oh, I wish I had been there." Six months after this conversation, I met Leticia, who told me that the family had changed a lot. Liisa had become more active and no longer talked about suicidal thoughts. Natalia, on the other hand, had become more anxious and was working on her own psychological concerns. Cristof had received support from a speech therapist and Liisa from the city's social services so that she could occasionally manage her own affairs without Cristof. Leticia said that in their conversations, they often asked each other what Jaakko would have said about this and that. This, of course, felt very nice because after the conversation I felt that the meeting had been very important to me. And apparently also for the family.

After the meeting, when we talked to the seminar audience, one psychiatrist wanted to say that he had never seen anything like this encounter. I assume he was referring both to the way the discussion was conducted and to the strong feelings that emerged and the open sharing of those feelings. In traditional psychiatric care, the expectation is that clinicians are neutral and do not share their own emotional experiences. In the most severe mental health crises, it is very difficult to remain neutral and unemotional in dialogue meetings because we always participate in the dialogue as living and experiencing persons, personally, even when it comes to professional help.

The psychiatrist's comment is in fact one of the motivations for writing this book. Having worked dialogically myself more than 40 years, dialogicity in my own therapy is a given. But time and again, when people observe dialogical therapists' conversations, they often tell that it is new and different for them. At the same time, when I know from multiple studies that this approach produces the best treatment outcomes, it is worth opening up the dimensions of dialogical life, dialogical encounter and dialogical helping. In the next chapter, I will consider the change in the understanding of the human being brought about by dialogicity, no longer primarily an analysis of the patient's symptoms and their elimination, but a bold engagement with the human experience.

Reference

Seikkula, J., Alakare, B., & Aaltonen, J. (2011). The comprehensive open-dialogue approach (II). Long-term stability of acute psychosis outcomes in advanced community care: The Western Lapland project. *Psychosis, 3*, 192–204. https://doi.org/10.1080/17522439.2011.595819

Chapter 3
From Empiricism to a Humane View of Human Being

"I've never seen anything like this," said the psychiatrist after following an Open Dialogue therapy session. Such an encounter was very surprising for a practitioner orientating to the symptoms, it did not seem to fit with his previous approach to treatment. It is a different understanding of the human being. To understand the effectiveness of dialogical practice, it is important to open up more broadly the basic assumptions of our view of human beings. My first response to why dialog cures is that dialogical practice has made it possible to meet people in their own context, respecting their individuality. In a diagnosis-driven way of thinking, a human image is created which does not allow us to believe in the results of Open Dialogue, for example in the case of psychotic problems. Dialogical practice creates a new image of the human, in which the best care is to accept people's emotional experiences rather than to eliminate psychological symptoms or change the family. While treatment recommendations tend to give generalizable and consistent guidelines, in a dialogical understanding of the human, each new encounter and each new dialogue creates a new reality, always for the first time. The mind is born in the flow of life.

Treatment Guidelines Are Based on a Strange Image of the Human Being

The promising results of dialogical practice confirm the assumption that, in a dialogical approach, we open the door to a new understanding of both problem-solving and the human being. In psychiatric discourse, there is little reflection on our understanding of human life. The person is assumed to be the embodiment of the differences between the mean scores of the treatment and control groups in clinical trials. If, for example, antidepressant medication achieves a faster recovery from depressive symptoms compared to no treatment, it is concluded that this result confirms that

J. Seikkula, *Why Dialogue Does Cure*,
https://doi.org/10.1007/978-3-031-91294-8_3

depression is a brain imbalance that requires medication to stimulate serotonin production.

Psychiatric practice based on evidence-based medicine treatment guidelines has not solved the problems of how to develop the most adequate care. Unfortunately, the worst situation is in the care of patients with the most severe mental health crises (such as schizophrenia). Reading the guidelines, one cannot avoid the thought that they very deliberately avoid Open Dialogue studies. After all, these studies have repeatedly shown out-of-this-world treatment results compared to conventional treatment. The question that worries me is: Why there is a refusal to take these results into account? The reason often given is that the results of studies cannot be included in treatment guidelines because they are not based on experimental research designs and there is no control group. These arguments are not true, as the results of Open Dialogue treatment have been compared with conventional psychiatric treatment (Chap. 1).

The symptoms-oriented view of humans seems to be very different from the humanistic conception of man that emerges in dialogical practice. Actually, one part of the problem is that there is no concept of human, or at least it is not made conscious. This is stated in the criteria for the guidelines in Finland, which state that ideological studies are not to be included in the recommendations. In the United Kingdom, the other line has been taken. There, the name used for the corresponding treatment recommendations is NICE, Treatment of excellence guidelines of best practice. The NICE recommendations also include a lot of research on psychotherapy studies and the qualitative dimensions of treatment.

In the empiricist view of man, the essence of man is defined in terms of his classifiable qualities. Classified attributes must be relatively stable for classifications to make sense. Naturally, the permanence of classifications is strengthened if biological, embodied factors can be found to underlie them. However, studies based mainly on comparing averages of the results obtained by different treatment groups and drawing conclusions from them will never be able to capture the actual characteristics of each individual. The outcome of a group, or more precisely the difference between the mean of the group under study and the mean of the control group, does not tell us anything about the scores obtained by an individual patient. Another problem comes from the fact that no comparison group is categorically mutually exclusive. Thus, conclusions about differences between some groups are drawn by comparing the mean scores of these groups at, say, the start of treatment and 1 year after the start of treatment. In most studies, with the exception of those on the Open Dialogue model of care, the variation in outcome within the two groups being compared is very similar. A statistically significant difference between two groups can occur if about 25% of the results in one group are outside the range of the comparison group. In practice, this means that 75% of the results in each group are within the same range. Thus, by far the majority of patients in the experimental group participating in the study have not shown any result that differs from the control group. Nevertheless, it is concluded that the result applies to all those in this group, although in fact most of the results in the different groups are within the same range. Thus, for example, the recommendation is made that all psychotic patients should be on medication for psychosis, even if only 25% of patients score better on a symptom measure than those not on medication.

Weak External Validity of Empirical Research

The importance of experimental controlled trials is stressed to arrive at universal treatment recommendations. This approach to research policy has led to a distortion of the emphasis on scientific research, as the results of controlled trials do not reflect the actual practice of treatment. In research parlance, their external validity is weak. Let me give one example of the shortcomings that can arise from this.

The treatment guidelines talk about evidence from studies. The most reliable evidence is defined as a study that compares one treatment method in a controlled way with another method or with a situation in which the treatment of one group is not specified. When a patient enters treatment, the study randomly assigns them to either a treatment group or a control group that does not receive the treatment being studied. In such a controlled setting, it is considered important that all other treatments are the same. To allow comparison between groups, the aim is to give everyone in each group the same dose of the treatment in question. This setting in itself is very problematic because in everyday practice patients do not receive the same dose of treatment, but the amount appropriate to each situation according to their own plan (an optimistic assumption that each has a plan). Some patients need to see their doctor more often, for example, because they have difficulty finding the right medication.

There are also many other problems with controlled experimental designs. It is very interesting that psychiatric researchers are aware of this, but despite this, the same policy continues to be applied in making treatment recommendations. Professor Jari Tiihonen, a professor of psychiatry, is perhaps the best-known international advocate of drug therapy in the treatment of psychosis. He also tends to give very one-sided interpretations of research findings. However, in an article (Taylor et al., 2012), he was also quoting as saying that

> Randomized controlled trials measure the effectiveness of (treatment) methods, but the experimental design affects the generalizability of the results in the 'real world', especially because of high dropout rates, short follow-up periods, and selection bias (…) Dropout rates even in very short follow-up studies of psychiatric drug treatment can be as high as 70% or 80%, making it difficult to interpret the results. In addition, large multicenter studies are very expensive to conduct, making them very difficult to initiate.

In fact, the authors point out that almost none of the arguments in favor of experimental research designs are true. Research results cannot be generalized to a real treatment situation ("real world") because of the high attrition rate required by a controlled trial design, the short follow-up time for treatment outcomes, and the selection of patients for the trial create a research bias, a bias effect on the trial. They also point to the fact that, for example, there is huge attrition in drug treatment trials. It may be that only 20% complete a trial. Interestingly, they also point out that large, controlled trials are very expensive to conduct, which limits in particular long-term follow-up. Researchers know that it is very difficult to obtain research funding for clinical mental health research and to recruit external researchers. Thus, the vast majority of research about psychosocial interventions is conducted by those who have developed the treatment model in their own environment. This actually helps the application of research findings, as the researchers are directly involved in treatment practice and have a better understanding of the relevance of the research findings. The external validity of the research is increased.

Do You Need Antipsychotic Medication?

The big difference between Open Dialogue and the effectiveness of conventional psychiatric treatment has puzzled me. One dimension seems to be that conventional treatment emphasizes the importance of neuroleptic medication, which is almost automatically initiated in the event of psychotic problems. Open Dialogue treatment, on the other hand, emphasizes that it is very important to select patients who really need medication. In this case, <20% were receiving antipsychotic medication at the beginning of treatment and, even after 19 years, much fewer than in conventional treatment. However, the results of the treatment were the opposite: those who automatically took medication had a much worse outcome than those who abstained or stopped taking medication. I have tried to understand this paradox by looking at long-term follow-up studies of neuroleptics. And I have repeatedly found problems with studies that justify automatic antipsychotic treatment. Let me give one example.

Taylor et al.'s response to the major problem of controlled experiments is to emphasize the importance of observational studies. Observational studies, for example, use national treatment statistics to monitor the treatment of patients in their natural environment without a specific research project during treatment. Indeed, a large group of Finnish psychiatry professors have carried out an internationally renowned project on the role of drug therapy in the treatment of patients with schizophrenia. This study has become almost canonical in the treatment guidelines for various countries, and the importance of neuroleptic therapy is emphasized with reference to this study.

Here is a description of their research (Tiihonen et al., 2009). Later, I will analyze the conclusions drawn from the results of the study. I have selected relevant parts of the text of their article:

> Finnish national statistics were used to determine the cause of death of 66,881 patients in relation to the total population (5.2 million) between 1996 and 2006, and this data was combined with the use of antipsychotic medication. We measured total mortality of schizophrenia patients in outpatient care in relation to antipsychotic medication use.
>
> Although the proportion of second-generation antipsychotics increased from 13% to 64% during the follow-up period, the gap in default age did not narrow between patients with schizophrenia and the general population (…). Long-term use of any antipsychotic (7–11 years) was associated with lower mortality than non-users (…) A total of 84 patients

> died during the follow-up period. The mortality rate of non-medicated patients was 10 times higher than that of medicated patients. 75 non-medicated patients died (3362 person-years) and nine medicated patients (4664 person-years). 26 non-medicated patients died by suicide compared to one medicated patient.

These quotes sum up the essential message, although I have not included all the technical information about the significance of the statistical values.

The Research Design Does Not Justify the Conclusions Drawn

So, the results seem very clear, don't they? Of course, this is also the unanimous conclusion of the authors of the study: neuroleptic medication is needed to prevent an increase in mortality rates. A closer look at the study report reveals its fundamental flaws. The study has also attracted widespread international criticism. De Hert et al. (2010) identified a number of problems with the study design and the selection of the patient population followed in the study. According to them:

> There is no information on the following variables: family status, diagnosis of alcohol and drug use, socioeconomic status, healthy life factors, detailed information on heart problems, and risk assessment information in general. As suicide occurs at an earlier stage of treatment, it has a very systematic effect on the study population, which makes the complex statistical methods used unjustified. Rather, confirmatory sensitivity analysis could have been performed equally well by matching all antipsychotic treatment groups to duration of illness.

When I read the study, I was looking for an answer to the question of whether the groups in the study were comparable. In other words, is the group that took medication similar to the group that did not take medication in terms of background variables and treatment experiences? To my surprise, I could not find any description of the groups in the study report. However, this is the most elementary principle of comparative statistical research. Now we have no idea on what other variables the difference between the groups might be based.

De Hert et al. continue their own criticism: "Tiihonen and colleagues report that 18,914 schizophrenia patients have not received any antipsychotic medication during the follow-up period (7.8 years) (146,930 person-years). It seems highly unlikely that 28.2% of patients would not have used antipsychotic medication or would not have been readmitted to hospital during the follow-up period. Previous studies by the same authors in smaller study populations have reported that patients had used antipsychotic medication at some point during follow-up (49% and 96%), and 21% of them had been readmitted during a shorter follow-up period (3.6 years). Another Finnish study reported that despite a reduction in hospital admissions, less than 4% were not receiving treatment (Salokangas et al., 2002). Finally, since in-hospital medication use was not taken into account, it was not included in this study."

So, they say there is a problem with the statistics presented in the study because quite different figures have been reported in the past on medication use, hospital admissions, and hospital use in general.

Knowing the Finnish psychiatric hospital treatment practice, it is safe to assume that all patients who have been hospitalized have been prescribed antipsychotic medication during their hospitalization. However, the use of medication during hospitalization has not been taken into account at all, but only medication after hospitalization. While the average length of hospitalization was initially 50 days, it is likely that almost all patients have been taking medication for at least 2 months. However, the study by Tiihonen et al. reports that 28.2% of all patients were in the non-medication group. In addition, the study did not report any new hospitalizations. However, around 70% of psychotic patients have recurrent hospitalizations, in which case they have also used medication.

The number of people not taking medication is therefore not correct. All—or almost all—patients have used antipsychotic medication, but some of them have not continued to use it in outpatient care after hospitalization. I believe that all those who have started taking medication have been recommended to continue taking antipsychotic medication after hospitalization. The majority of patients have acted on the recommendation (77.8%), but a smaller proportion have not (28.2%), so we have no information on the reasons for discontinuing the recommended medication. We also do not know what has happened during a relapsed hospitalization.

De Hert et al. also found problems with the reliability of the reported mortality rates compared to previous studies. They note that when comparing mortality rates with other studies, the Tiihonen et al. study shows very low rates in the chlorpromazine patient group (the most common antipsychotic). In this study, the mortality rate was 5.69 per 1000 people per year. In other studies, it was 8.5, 11.3, and 12.5 (Taylor et al., 2009; Munro et al., 1999; Meltzer et al., 2003). They say that it remains to be seen whether the low mortality rate is real or linked to the chosen study design. They see the chosen research methods as very biased.

Two types of serious problems emerge from the study. Firstly, the validity of the statistical figures has been criticized because they are so different from previous statistics. Furthermore, the researchers do not provide any information on how the selection of this particular study group has influenced these statistics. Secondly, the study groups do not actually tell the difference, which is what the authors of the study stated they wanted to report. These groups are not the medication-taking group versus the non-medication-taking group. The "real world" groups are the group that took and continued the recommended medication versus the group that stopped the recommended medication. There is a large body of research evidence that abruptly stopping antipsychotic medication increases the risk of new psychosis and other withdrawal symptoms.

This kind of comparison is also very interesting and important because it would include the actual practice of care, that is, the actual care situations, the "real world." Now researchers are drawing conclusions about things that cannot be drawn from this study. Although the stated aim was to do "real world" research, in the end the research did not.

Where does this indifference to the basics of scientific research come from? I do not think it is ignorance since they are all professors who are well versed in research methods. It could be that researchers are just careless and think that these issues are not that important to consider because the importance of antipsychotic medication is taken for granted. So, it cannot be questioned. It may also be that they are reporting the results of the research in a purposive way. Whitaker (2020) did an in-depth analysis of studies showing that antipsychotic medication prolongs life expectancy. In the Tiihonen group's studies, he cites many of the problems with the research methodology outlined above and suggests that the purpose of these studies was not so much to investigate the role of antipsychotic use in patients' lives, but to find a rationale for long-term use of antipsychotics.

Results of an Externally Valid Study Suggest Risks of Drug Treatment

In another study in Finland, it was used the register data to make a comparison (Bergström et al., 2020), taking into account the shortcomings that affect the reliability of the Tiihonen group's results. The results were largely opposite to the conclusions drawn by that study. In fact, it was found that long-term use of antipsychotic medication was associated with prolonged treatment, entrance into ongoing disability, and increased mortality.

These results are in line with those already published earlier by Joukamaa et al. (2006). They studied the life course and mortality of patients with schizophrenia from a cohort of all people born in Northern Finland in 1966. The mortality of schizophrenia patients who took medication, especially more than one medication, was significantly higher than those who did not take medication. They found:

> During 17 years of follow-up, 39/99 patients with schizophrenia died. When this was related to age and sex, the relative mortality risk between schizophrenia patients and others was 2.84 and 2.25 when further related to somatic disease, blood pressure, cholesterol, body mass index, smoking, physical activity, alcohol consumption and education. The number of neuroleptics used at baseline was associated with an increased risk of mortality. Relative risk was 2.50 for every 1 additional neuroleptic drug, when adjusted for age, sex, somatic disease and other potential risk factors for early mortality.

They reported that 24 patients (34%) were not taking medication. They were more often male, less likely to be on a disability pension, more likely to have recovered from their illness, and had a better overall clinical situation. If the patient had not been hospitalized in the previous 5 years, they were more likely to have stopped taking antipsychotic medication without readmission. They concluded that some patients with schizophrenia do better without permanent antipsychotic medication.

This study of the Northern Finland cohort is much more reliable than a comparison of national statistics. Especially when the comparison of national statistics includes measures to select the study population. Of course, the data for the Northern Finland cohort is much smaller, which makes it more challenging to predict the persistence of the results for Finland as a whole. It is interesting that the Tiihonen study makes no reference to the Joukamaa study. I wonder if this is a political statement and if it is not so important to scrupulously observe the ethical principles of scientific research if one can benefit from one's own bias.

Be that as it may, when I read this kind of sloppiness or deliberate manipulation of data, my assumption is that the standard of research is not so stable. A particular problem is its low level of external validity. When studies are conducted under laboratory conditions, no information is obtained about the effects of the treatment in a real-life situation. And when those who insist on conducting a study that corresponds to the actual treatment situation start to conduct an observational study, they seem to manipulate the study groups and draw conclusions contrary to the study design.

The Finnish treatment guidelines create a picture of a person as a collection of the symptoms he or she is experiencing. And treatment is then about eliminating these symptoms in the most effective way possible. *The risk of this way of thinking is that it is not accompanied by an understanding of the meaning of the symptoms and their relationship to the life of the individual.*

Understanding Comes from Dialogue: Not from Naming a Diagnosis

Dialogical knowledge is created in relationships and is useful in each interaction. *Transferring this knowledge to another situation requires a new dialogue in which we can understand the new meaning of things.* A colleague of mine once said, when we were thinking about this, "That sounds like a dialogical jungle. So, we always need a new dialogue to understand the meaning of something, and that can only be understood by the participant in the dialogue?" he asked. For me too, his comment was an insight I had not been able to put into words before. That's exactly it. In that conversation with my colleague, we were considering whether the decisions made in a therapy meeting for a patient in a hospital ward could be binding on those who were not involved in the meeting. We have often found in the hospital that it is very difficult to make treatment decisions binding on others. I assume that the difficulty of this issue is linked to that very insight. *It is only by engaging in dialogue and creating a shared experience that we can understand it in a profound way that guides our actions.* Making a diagnosis, for example, is not yet an understanding, it is only the discovery of some things and the classification of their coherence.

An empirical understanding of knowledge starts from a different set of assumptions about the relationship between reality and the knowledge about it. For example, it is assumed that the causes of a patient's illness can be explained unambiguously by studies comparing this group of patients with those who are not ill. These comparisons aim to provide a stable body of knowledge that is generalizable to all circumstances. When several such studies are carried out on the same subject, a systematic analysis can then be carried out and, on the basis of this analysis, treatment recommendations can be made for the disease in question.

Treatment guidelines based on this kind of generalizable research have been made since the early 1990s. That is a very long time. There has been no long-term follow-up of their impact, so we don't know much about the impact of treatment guidelines. The 19-year follow-up study I quoted in the first chapter and the comparison between the open dialogue in Western Lapland and the rest of Finland is probably the only long-term comparison of psychosis treatment. The results of conventional treatment have not evolved. In some situations, treatment guidelines based on laboratory tests can even be harmful by producing recommendations that may have a basis in research, but which in fact prevent the patient from being confronted in a way that would increase his or her resources and those of his or her loved ones in crisis.

Dialogical Human Image Depicts a Living Human Being

A dialogical view of the human being is much more in tune with the true nature of life. One of the great thinkers of dialogism is Professor Ivana Markova, who has a university career in Scotland. One of the most important works in her rich output is the book *Dialogical Mind* (Markova, 2016), in which she outlines a dialogical view of the human being. The dialogical view of the human person is in some respects quite different from the view of the human person as a set of fixed attributes that determine our perceptions, behavior, emotions, and ultimately our psychological symptoms. As I write this chapter, her book is very much on my mind.

The dialogical conception of the human being is interactive. The human mind is built in and from relationships, and thus cannot be a permanent construct of qualities. Every relationship shapes the human mind, every interaction situation always creates a new challenge. All interaction situations are unique so that change is always inevitable. We cannot enter the same stream twice. Helping people in mental health and other crises opens up a whole new world of possibilities. All relationships and interactions can be helpful because they create new unique meanings.

It is difficult to put the dialogical approach of helping into a specific category. Similarly, the philosophical view of humanity outlined in this book does not as such fit into any particular school or orientation. Initially, when developing the dialogical way of working in the 1980s and 1990s, it was very important for me to frame the reality of therapeutic work in terms of social constructionism, because it allowed me to abandon the search for objective truth. Before that, when I studied the systemic model of family therapy in the early 1980s, I was trying to find a systemic approach to the family problem. Systemic family therapy sought to determine the function of the symptom of the family member who came to see me as a patient in terms of family homeostasis. The idea was that there was a correct explanation that the therapists had to find. The family therapists' intervention focused on the family interaction system rather than on the family members as individuals.

The writings of Kenneth Gergen and John Shotter were particularly important for family therapy. They summed up even more poignantly how we construct our reality socially, as if between people. It is not the objective meaning of a problem that is central, but the meanings we give to it in social interaction. Thus, for example, psychotic problems cannot be objectively defined in only one way, but from our point of view, the phenomenon itself always becomes different. We can see a medical dimension to psychotic behavior because we can describe a particular type of behavior as a diagnostic category. However, diagnostic manuals are descriptions of syndromes, not descriptions of the basis of the problem itself.

Indeed, psychosis cannot be understood in just one way, but it has many different meanings depending on our perspective. We can see a lot of social dimensions in psychotic behavior because it directly affects the individual's social relationships. The experiential aspect of psychosis also opens up an interesting perspective, because often the person behaving psychotically perceives external reality differently from those around him or her. We can also see a strong ethical aspect to the psychotic problem, as it allows the community to exercise power over the other person by forcing them into treatment against their will. The physical dimensions of psychosis, such as its neurobiological links, have also been much described. Empirical science seeks to find one correct perspective that defines the fundamental nature of psychosis (or any other disorder). It too, of course, accepts the existence of all the different dimensions, but they are subordinate to the correct explanation. In recent decades, psychiatry has been dominated by the neurobiological model of explanation, which sees mental disorders as structural problems of brain function.

The neurobiological explanation of man and man's problems is very limited, as it gives room for only a small part of all approaches to defining man. It monopolizes one view as the correct one. The human brain is always part of the interaction between the different parts of the human body, and the human body is always part of the interaction with external physical reality. These parts—internal and external—do not remain the same but are constantly changing. No more can human psychological characteristics and thereby human psychological problems be reduced to a specific area of brain activity or dysfunction.

John Shotter was particularly interested in how and what kind of information we create about our reality. According to him, the knowledge that guides our actions (Shotter, 1993) becomes different depending on whether we know something about an object outside ourselves, or whether our knowledge is constructed in relation to the object of knowledge. Empirical science and the recommendations for current care based on it assume that it is possible to create generalized knowledge about the object of study and thus provide treatment guidelines that are valid in different situations. This is what knowing-about is. Another kind of knowing is when we experience, together with the subject of our observations, their lives. For this Shotter uses the term knowing-from-within. On the basis of this distinction, one might consider, for example, the difference between the diagnosis we make by observing from the outside and the diagnosis we make by interacting with our clients. Diagnoses are seen as objective descriptions of the object of diagnosis. It is important to find just the right diagnosis. To enable this, different symptoms are accurately described and classified. In most cases, it is these symptoms that are then used to find the correct diagnosis.

In knowing-from-within, the diagnosis is made in the relationship that is happening right now. Thus, the observation in the discussion in the therapy meeting that the person is talking about something that I do not perceive, allows us to assume that he or she is having psychotic experiences. This knowledge, in turn, influences the progress of the conversation. It does not determine it, but it influences it in many ways. This is different when trying to define an objective diagnosis, where it is often important to define the person's experience as psychotic, ill, and to tell him or her this by helping to reality-test him or her. So, he or she can be told that what you are telling them is not true but is part of your psychotic illness. Thus, the outside observer has done his job.

But by knowing-from-within, we become part of the person's life and experience. This is what makes it possible to help. So in the dialogue of the Open Dialogue therapy meeting, we do not use reifying comments like the one above, but we try to encourage the telling of more stories about his/her experience in order to understand more not only about the psychosis itself but also about his/her life. Psychosis as a phenomenon becomes very different from trying to find just the right diagnosis. Our actions determine our perceptions, and our perceptions determine the way we interact with the person who needs help.

Dialogue and the Copernican Revolution in Philosophy

However, understanding the role of the observer in the construction of our reality is not at all a constructionist invention. As early as the 1700s in philosophy, Immanuel Kant argued that knowledge of reality could not be achieved by the mere reproduction of sensory perceptions, but that knowledge was formed by a method of rule-based synthesis. According to him, causal explanations of natural laws emerge in our minds through interaction with reality outside ourselves. This is what Kant called the Copernican revolution in philosophy, referring to the astronomer Copernicus, who broke with the prevailing view of the Earth as the center of the universe.

Kant's work has been a point of departure for a great many philosophical trends of the time, which have had in common the continuation of his theory of the centrality of the human mind in describing reality. In the early 1900s, several key philosophers such as Martin Heidegger, Ludwig Wittgenstein, and Ernst Cassirer all described the central role of language in our perception of reality (Eilenberger, 2019). In this respect, Wittgenstein's work became particularly pivotal when, in another book, he argued that our worldview is constructed through the use of language in everyday life. We live in language games that define the boundaries of our reality, he said. Beyond a general philosophical understanding of knowledge, this insight of Wittgenstein's is revolutionary and goes straight to the heart of the dialogical view of the human being. The theory of knowledge is not something that exists in general and determines our sensory perceptions and reasoning, but knowledge is constructed through the use of language in practical life situations, pragmatically. This view also comes very close to the specific focus of the dialogical style of therapy, in that we no longer focus our attention so much on the stories that clients in therapy tell about their lives and their reality, but more on the interactional event in which we use language to describe reality. It is interesting that Wittgenstein did little to describe this relational dimension of language use. From a dialogical point of view, the relation becomes the most important, because the way we use language and the way we create our reality in it always takes place in some relation. We are therefore constantly in a relationship of influence and agency because the language we use is responded to by the people we are with.

As a description of the dialogue, what I wrote above is clumsy. When we describe phenomena, we use abstract language, which is very limited compared to the richness of the language spoken in practice. In the abstract description of language, we cannot capture the rich, multicolored flow of conversation, in which we cannot distinguish between the influencer and the influenced.

Reality Is Born at the Boundary

How have these different descriptions of life related to the development of a dialogical practice of care? I was part of the team that started to develop the practice of open therapy meetings in the Keropudas Hospital in Tornio in the early 1980s. In an open therapy meeting, therefore, everyone involved in care participates from the beginning, without prior planning, in a common, open discussion. We immediately realized that language was a key factor in this new family-centered way of working, where everything was discussed openly together with the patient and his or her family. There was an unexpected tension because we were working in an environment where the starting point was to diagnose and define the patient's symptoms and the treatment methods needed to overcome them, but in fact, we were already working in a different culture of care, in open therapy meetings, where each time a new reality and a new care plan were created. It was impossible to follow a treatment plan that had been drawn up previously because a good discussion in a new meeting could bring a whole new understanding of the family's situation. We had created a new paradigm.

I worked hard to understand this tension. First, I read a lot of philosophical literature on language and the meaning of language. For example, Hintikka (1982) has done a lot of philosophical research on the relationship between language and reality. His descriptions are philosophical and relevant within philosophy, but they were difficult to apply to the everyday language user. It is interesting to repeat his description here, however, because he has criticized Wittgenstein's description of language as a universal phenomenon. That is, as if our reality is constructed in language, and it is not possible to transcend the boundaries of language. Hintikka, however, is more critical of Wittgenstein's interpreters because he says Wittgenstein is misinterpreted (Pihlström, 1998). According to Hintikka, a better understanding of the relationship between language and the world comes when we understand that language is a calculus, a means by which we describe reality. In such an understanding of language, we can also find a truth that is not tied to language's descriptions of reality.

This distinction and reflection, interesting in itself, did little to provide answers for understanding the phenomena generated by the practice of therapy meetings. Philosophical descriptions seemed to be mostly very distant from the need to apply the language of practical life. Similarly, the focus of philosophical descriptions on the reality of individual perceptions and experiences, as described above, seems to be of little help in a relationship-centered world. Such a view of the human person is also limited because it fails to consider life as a relational flow. With good intentions, one may build a picture of the human being that misses something that is absolutely essential to the overall picture.

In this situation, I came across Mikhail Bakhtin's dialogicity and polyphony. And this relational description of life seemed to hit the mark immediately. When open therapy meetings started to be organized at Keropudas Hospital in 1984, they were an immediate success. They seemed to give patients many new opportunities. At the same time, we also began to have repeated and unexpected confusing experiences where the patient's recovery only began after us as clinicians had changed.

If we look at this from a more distant perspective, we can consider that we, as caregivers, are working according to the traditional psychiatric model of care and also according to the systemic family therapy model. Systemic family therapy is, in this respect, to some extent in line with the empiricist view of human nature, because it assumes that the family functions as a system that obeys certain laws, which must be defined and then modified by the interventions of family therapists. There is one correct definition of a family system and a family therapy intervention based on it.

In psychiatric care, a similar mindset is followed. First, the patient's problems are identified, and specific treatment plans are made for them, which are then followed upon. This model works well in many areas of medicine. For example, if a patient is found to have elevated blood sugar levels, analyses are carried out to determine whether he or she may have diabetes and specific treatment methods are followed to manage diabetes. The focus of treatment is on the patient's symptoms and the treatment measures to address them.

In our open care practice, two different conceptions of the human being and two different paradigms collided. When we started our open therapy meetings, we continued to act according to the model we had learned as symptom-relieving providers of the patient according to the care plan. In repeated confusing impasse situations, change began with a change of us as providers, not in the patient or family. This change opened the way to better outcomes. Such a reality is not part of empiricist worldview-based care, where caregivers' interventions bring about a change in the patient's symptoms. Based on repeated similar observations, I began to use the term 'boundary system' to describe the fact that an autonomous system of action seemed to emerge at the boundary between the family and the hospital, which followed its own laws without regard to the care plan. The effort to be therapeutic did not yet change anything, but the events themselves did. The idea of a boundary system was a compromise between systemic and interactional thinking. I thought that the system was important, not as a permanent description of a set of interactions, but as something that was always being constructed in each interaction. This observation, with all its limitations, helped to develop a new model of care. It was also the basis for my dissertation on how this "boundary system" works when a care team meets a patient referred to the hospital with his family at the first therapy meeting (Seikkula, 1991, see also Chap. 9).

In boundary systems, we often found ourselves in situations where we did not understand what was happening. As I said above, I tried to look for a solution in philosophers' descriptions of the meaning of language without finding an answer. In one discussion, as we were reflecting on recurring challenging situations, one of the participants in the discussion began to recall his student days and told me about Erkki Peuranen, a professor of Russian at the University of Jyväskylä, who was very interested in Mikhail Bakhtin's work. He said that my descriptions reminded him of these texts by Peuranen and referred to an article published in Kulttuurivihkot magazine (Peuranen, 1980). When I opened the article by Erkki Peuranen, I was amazed. Although the content of the article was Bakhtin's description of the polyphony and dialogicity of Dostoyevsky's novel world, it described our experiences in psychiatric hospital therapy meetings in great detail. Peuranen opened with a brief description of how Bakhtin thought that the world of Dostoevsky's novels was very special because in it all the characters in the novel seem to have their own truth, which no one else can deny. Interestingly, Markova speaks of the characters in Dostoevsky's novels as anti-heroes, because they may be murderers or otherwise break the rules of society. But nevertheless, they carry their own voice in a dialogical relationship with others. Bakhtin calls such a novel a polyphonic novel. There are always as many voices as there are speakers. Since no one else can contradict the truth of one character, the only way for the story to develop is to seek dialogue with other characters in the novel. In this dialogue, each character finds an answer for himself and, in his inner dialogue, creates his own identity. Life is thus a jungle of voices, and in dialogue with others, one understands one's own starting point.

The description was a disturbingly accurate account of our experiences in open therapy meetings. It was impossible to identify a single most important character or to categorize the most important problem, as all participants in the therapy meeting seemed to have their own understanding of the current crisis and problem. And that's not all. While we often felt we were losing control in the implementation of treatment plans, Bakhtin also described how the writer of polyphonic novels loses control over his or her characters in the novel. The writer's only chance of survival is to try to enter into dialogue with his or her characters. In this type of polyphonic novel, it is no longer possible to identify one voice as the right one and, with the help of the other characters in the novel, carry this hero through the story in the direction the author wants. This was exactly our experience at the therapy meetings. It is no longer possible for us as providers to control the understanding and actions of the participants in therapy meetings, but we are left only with the option of adapting to the voices of the family and the rest of the network.

Philosophy Reaches Only Part of Our Human Image

Understanding the phenomena of a new view of the human being and the practice of dialogical therapy through philosophical descriptions did not initially shed much light on the subject. Although philosophy is generally regarded as a progressive phenomenon, it can also have very old-fashioned elements that hinder understanding. Thus, in an attempt to analyze a concept, one may unknowingly accept very pathological descriptions of a person in need. This has often been seen in philosophical descriptions of schizophrenia.

Fortunately for us, there have also been other currents in philosophy in general and phenomenology in particular, which see man as a bodily participant in the flow of life, and as an active shaper of this flow of life. This understanding was already cultivated by Maurice Merleau-Ponty and, long before him, by the American philosopher and psychologist William James. In addition to these, philosophy has become increasingly interested in embodiment and its study, and this has also given rise to new active descriptions of embodied social knowledge. Much new neuroscience and brain research has been incorporated into this knowledge.

Dialogical practice builds a shared experience, where there is not one actor and one subject. In dialogue, participants are constantly constructing a shared reality in which everyone interacts with each other. Merleau-Ponty opened up the understanding that bodily perceptions always take place in interactive situations. However, not always necessarily in direct interaction, as the other party can also be a building, a work of art or other non-breathing elements of reality. It was also important for Merleau-Ponty to understand the construction of a reciprocal relationship independent of language, alongside language.

All this has also enriched our understanding of the potential for dialogical processes. For example, in order to make use of the results of brain research, it is important to understand the kind of person to whom the different phenomena of brain activity are related. If we think of brain function as the basis of human functioning, brain research as a means of identifying the causes of human functioning, and brain research as a means of identifying the causes of mental disorders, we create an image of a predetermined human being and see problematic situations as pathological phenomena. Thus, for example, the description of schizophrenia does not arouse much interest in the person himself, because his pathology is thought to determine him.

The dialogical image of humans of humans is interested in all people in the here-and-now interaction in which everyone participates with their whole body—including their brain—but now it is humanity itself and the uniqueness of the human being that generates the interest in the other. The most important knowledge comes not from the results of brain research but from our shared reality and the meanings that emerge from it.

To build a valid and adequate knowledge of the human being, it is necessary to bring the philosophical attitude described here to research. Shotter (1993) talked a lot about the fact that science should not strive for objective knowledge of the same kind, but that all knowledge comes from the use of knowledge. He used the term argumentative knowledge for this. Ivana Markova spoke of the emergence of important knowledge in the tension of the I—Other relationship. So, there are several ways of talking about how we create valid knowledge about a person, taking him or her bodily into account every moment as a participant, respondent, initiator, or reactor in a reciprocal interaction.

The study of the scientific tradition has described two dimensions of scientific knowledge, mythos and logos. Mythos knowledge is knowledge generated in stories, which naturally requires participation in situations where stories are shared. The telling of one story gives rise to new stories. Logos knowledge, on the other hand, is generated by logical reasoning, by brain activity. We try to discover the basic nature of the phenomenon under study by correct reasoning through the analysis of the different parts of the phenomena. Often this kind of knowledge is close to experimental research. Narrative knowledge, on the other hand, arises closer to the life event itself. This opens an interesting question about the kind of research data we need to understand and develop dialogical practices.

References

Bergström, T., Seikkula, J., Alakare, B., Mäki, P., Köngäs-Saviaro, P., Taskila, J. J., et al. (2018). The family-oriented open dialogue approach in the treatment of first-episode psychosis: Nineteen-year outcomes. *Psychiatry Research, 270*, 168–175.

Bergström, T., Taskila, J., Alakare, B., Köngäs-Saviaro, P., Miettunen, J., & Seikkula, J. (2020). Five-year cumulative exposure to antipsychotic medication after first-episode psychosis and its association with 19-year outcomes. *Schizophrenia Bulletin Open*. https://doi.org/10.1093/schizbullopen/sgaa050

De Hert, M., Correll, C., & Cohen, D. (2010). Do antipsychotic medications reduce or increase mortality in schizophrenia? A critical appraisal of the FIN-11 study. *Schizophrenia Research, 117*, 68–74.

Eilenberger, L. (2019). *Time of the magicians. The great decade of philosophy 1919 - 1929*. Penguin Books.

Hintikka, J. (1982). *Language and mind: Reviews on the philosophy of language and the theory of meaning*. Otava.

Joukamaa, M., Heliovaara, M., Knekt, P., Aromaa, A., Raitasalo, R., & Lehtinen, V. (2006). Schizophrenia, neuroleptic medication and mortality. *The British Journal of Psychiatry, 188*, 122–127.

Markova, I. (2016). *The dialogical mind. Common sense and ethics*. Cambridge University Press. https://doi.org/10.1017/CBO9780511753602

Meltzer, H. Y., Alphs, L., Green, A. I., Altamura, A. C., Anand, R., Bertoldi, A., Bourgeois, M., Chouinard, G., Islam, M. Z., Kane, J., Krishnan, R., Lindenmayer, J. P., Potkin, S., & International Suicide Prevention Trial Study Group. (2003). Clozapine treatment for suicidality in schizophrenia: International Suicide Prevention Trial (InterSePT). *Archives of General Psychiatry, 60*(1), 82–91.

Munro, J., O'Sullivan, D., Andrews, C., Arana, A., Mortimer, A., & Kerwin, R. (1999). Active monitoring of 12,760 clozapine recipients in the UK and Ireland. *British Journal of Psychiatry, 175*, 576–580.

Peuranen, E. (1980). Bahtinin sosiaalinen poetiikka. *Kulttuurivihkot, 1*, 17–27.

Pihlström, S. (1998). Jaakko Hintikka, Ludwig Wittgenstein and the dichotomy of philosophy in our century. *So & So, 3*(98), 38–48.

Salokangas, R., Honkonen, T., Stengård, E., & Koivisto, A. M. (2002). Mortality in chronic schizophrenia during decreasing number of psychiatric beds in Finland. *Schizophrenia Research, 54*(3), 265–275.

Seikkula, J. (1991). *The family-hospital boundary system* [Family-hospital boundary system in the social network. English summary]. Jyväskylä Studies in Education, Psychology and Social Research, 80.

Shotter, J. (1993). *Cultural politics of every day life. Social constructionism, rhetoric and knowing of the third kind.* Open University Press.

Taylor, D. M., Douglas-Hall, P., Olofinjana, B., Whiskey, E., & Thomas, A. (2009). Reasons for discontinuing clozapine: Matched, case-control comparison with risperidone long-acting injection. *The British Journal of Psychiatry, 194*(2), 165–167.

Taylor, M., Cavanagh, J., Hodgson, R., & Tiihonen, J. (2012). Examining the effectiveness of antipsychotic medication in first-episode psychosis. *Journal of Psychopharmacology, 26*, 27–32.

Tiihonen, J., Lönnqvist, J., Wahlbeck, K., Klaukka, T., Niskanen, L. Tanskanen, A. & Haukka J. (2009, July 13). *11-year follow-up of mortality in patients with schizophrenia: A population-based cohort study (FIN11 study)*. www.thelancet.com

Whitaker, R. (2020). *Do anti-psychotics protect against early death? A review of the evidence*. https://www.madinamerica.com/2020/05/do-antipsychotics-protect-against-early-death-a-review-of-the-evidence/

Chapter 4
Life Is a Stream of Participation: The Intersubjective Revolution

The second part of my answer to the question of why dialogue improves is to look more closely at the dialogical conception of the human being in the light of intersubjectivity. Dialogical practice embraces and draws on the latest intersubjective knowledge that humans are, from birth, active participants in interaction—rhythmically and bodily. The mind is born in relationships, and in these relationships, man is the constructor of his own development. The treatment of severe mental health crises should take into account the human being as a holistic bodily participant in a constantly evolving flow of interaction, a dialogue. When we understand the power of dialogue as a fundamental dimension of human life, we can be confident that even seemingly simple conversational methods are very helpful.

"Life Is To Participate in Dialogue"

As mentioned in the previous chapter, dialogicity opens up a new understanding of human life. In this chapter, I seek to deepen the contribution of intersubjectivity research, according to which the human mind emerges as embodied experience in our relationships, past and present. This is why working with families and networks is central to my work. In the next chapter (Chap. 5), I describe how family therapy has moved from seeking a single systemic description to understanding the polyphony of here-and-now interactions as embodied phenomena. And then in Chap. 6, I describe the embodied, relational mind based on the research that we have conducted with my research team. The human mind is dialogical. For Mikhail Bakhtin, human life is a continuous dialogue in which we participate with all our actions and our whole body. Dialogue becomes a value in itself because in dialogue we connect with each other and carry out our lives.

Although Bakhtin was a literary scholar and philosopher, he provides important guidance for psychotherapists: The aim of therapy is to create a dialogue in the here and now, because in a dialogue the person becomes himself for the first time. The

J. Seikkula, *Why Dialogue Does Cure*,
https://doi.org/10.1007/978-3-031-91294-8_4

dialogical understanding is different from the psychological description of the human being in terms of different personality traits. These aim at permanent descriptions. Such descriptions have also given rise to a number of psychotherapeutic orientations, which then provide guidelines for dealing with different personalities and different problems. Some have also incorporated brain research as part of the understanding of personality differences. Brain studies also provide a wealth of information that can be used in therapy. For example, many therapeutic approaches today draw on attachment theory, which suggests that our early attachment experiences influence our behavior in today's relationships. Close attachments, such as romantic love relationships, become particularly important. Specific therapeutic methods have been developed on the basis of different attachment experiences, such as in emotion-focused couples therapy. I take attachment theories here as an example because there is a lot of useful brain research on them currently. Different attachment experiences have been found to produce different brain patterns and even brain dysfunctions, which can then be corrected in psychotherapy (Hughes, 2015).

"Experience Is a Distinctive Set of Sensations"

Let's return to the dialogical description of man. Bakhtin was not the first thinker to open up the human experience as a here-and-now participation. One of those who, shortly before Bakhtin, did the bulk of his life's work was the American psychologist and philosopher William James, who studied the neural structure of human beings in animal experiments. In one of his most famous books from 1892, *Stream of Consciousness*, he noted:

> Our experiences are sensations of tendencies, and they are often so weak that we cannot name them at all (p. 254). Such sensations can serve as directional cues from thoughts that give rise to an acutely discriminating perception, even if no image created by the sense has any role to play in this (p. 253).

According to him, human experiences are tendentious sensations, most often not formed into explicit verbal stories, but into sensations of differences. It also opens up our understanding of emotions. According to James, emotions are sensations of the body. This can open up new meanings for psychotherapy, where we are used to thinking that the consultants verbalize their emotional experiences and then together with the therapist they give meaning to those experiences. But James draws our attention to the fact that most emotional experiences are just acute sensory images without words. According to Shotter (2011), James' descriptions of human experiences are not looking for repetitive patterns. Our experiences happen in the flow of life and rush forward so that by the time we start talking about an experience, we are already in another emotional experience. This emotional experience can, of course, arise from talking about that particular memory, which is then the basic idea of dialogical discussion. According to Shotter, James' description of experience is different from Gregory Bateson's description of systems, which, according to Bateson, create recurrent patterns of action. Bateson's theory has had a major influence on systemic family therapy, which seeks to identify the recurring patterns of the family system. Open Dialogue, on the other hand, sees the experiences of family members as unique to each situation.

The human mind is a dialogical process in which life-guiding meanings are created. American professor in psychiatry Siegel (2010) has become renowned for applying the knowledge of brain research to psychotherapy. He defined the human mind as "a communal and embodied process that regulates the flow of energy and information." As we saw, James described with surprising accuracy over a century ago how the human body works and creates sensations that then guide our choices and how we proceed. These are not really experiences, because they are not put into words, but they are often sensations that affect us strongly.

"Movement Is the First Language"

The description of the human mind as an embodied function has evolved a lot in the last couple of decades. The philosopher Maxine Sheet-Johnstone (2010) has been very interested in the cultural-historical school of psychology that originated in Russia, originally during the Soviet era. She is particularly interested in the neuropsychology of the psychologist Alexander Luria. Luria is generally regarded as the father of neuropsychology. Sheet-Johnstone's area of expertise has been dance and movement therapy. According to her, the human mind is born in movement. She stresses that the first language of man is the language of movement. Babies regulate their emotional experiences and communicate through their movements. The Russian psychologist Lev Vygotsky (1935/1982) created a description of language. According to him, language has three functions. Language is how we communicate; language is how we regulate our actions and language is how we think. If we think of a newborn baby, amazingly, two of those three basic functions of language are already in use by the baby. When we regulate our own actions, we are above all regulating our own emotional arousal. When a baby starts to sense discomfort in the stomach, we adults would say he is hungry, but the baby senses nothing of the sort because hunger is already a big inference from some bodily experience. But the baby senses discomfort, she starts making noises and moving her arms, legs, and body. With these movements, the baby regulates its own affective arousal. Gradually this develops into crying and more intense movements. This is usually—and hopefully—when the mother or father reacts and starts to comfort the baby and prepare food and eventually, through the satisfaction of food, the baby calms down. What was initially a regulation of one's own emotional arousal, that is, movements, vocalizations, and crying, becomes at the same time communication inviting mother or father to help her.

This is one of the most crucial experiences in life and illustrates well the concept of intersubjectivity: By her own movements and vocalizations, the baby invites the mother or father to regulate her emotional arousal. The Other becomes part of the regulation of his emotional arousal, the Other becomes part of the Self. From the beginning, life is a dialogue in which we seek an answer for ourselves. In this process, the baby begins to recognize herself and through many repetitions, her anticipation becomes stronger, and the father and mother become increasingly powerful inner voices in life. The baby also learns the differences between the parents, because the pacifying of the father and mother are not the same, but both can help. The baby, and the human being in general, is a collection of sounds that emerge from different relationship experiences through rhythmic synchrony. In this way of thinking, it is difficult to speak of the individual, because the psychic regulation always involves the other or the experience of the other as an inner voice. The boundary of the individual is not his skin, but the individual includes all the interpersonal relationships, the voices, of the life he experiences. The individual is therefore "intersubjective," constructed by relationships, rather than "intrasubjective," defined from within.

In his short career, Lev Vygotsky was a pioneer of a new kind of psychological thinking. In addition to the development of the emergence of language, he was very interested in how meanings or minds are created. According to him, we sense each other's emotional states in our collective actions. Describing his experiments with children, he noted:

> In our research on the connection between movement and motor activity and emotional processes, we found that the motor movement response is so embedded and inextricably part of the emotional process that it can serve as a reflective mirror, where it is literally possible to read the structure of the emotional process hidden from direct perception (Vygotsky, 1930, p. 31).

According to Vygotsky, we synchronize with each other in interaction situations so that our bodily functions begin to merge with the reactions of the other body. Through these bodily reactions, we can access the emotions we experience, even if we cannot directly perceive or name them. What is puzzling about Vygotsky's comment is that he identified this phenomenon in his own research in 1930, more than 60 years before anyone had talked about mirror neurons. In his descriptions, too, man as an agent in his relationships constructs himself and his language in an ever-evolving process of understanding himself in relation to others.

Surprisingly, the idea of this "new" image of man is not new, but we can assume that our attempt to create a new image of man and a new understanding of the human mind is based on a very strong scientific tradition in several disciplines. None of the scholars mentioned in this chapter consider the human being as a single property, the same constant agent, but all describe how, through our own bodily actions in interpersonal relationships, we create mind as an ever-flowing, rather than a constant, property.

Psychoanalyst Daniel Stern (2004) is known as a researcher and practitioner of baby communication research. Empowered by the intersubjective view of the human being, he found this to be a revolutionary insight into the development of the human mind. According to him, the human mind develops through sensorimotor activity in relation to other human minds. In this statement, he is very close to what Vygotsky said about the emotional process being related to the motor activity of the body, the movement.

The Baby Is the Author of Her Own Growth

The study of intersubjectivity has broadened our understanding of the human mind. For a long time, the Western view of man was dominated by Sigmund Freud's idea that a baby is psychologically empty at birth. According to this theory, the psychic birth of a human being does not occur until about 6 months of age (Mahler et al., 1973). Before then, the baby lives in an autistic world of experience in symbiosis with her mother. A similar description of psychic development was supported by the Swiss developmental psychologist Jean Piaget, who also had a major influence on the Western view of the human being. This conception of the human being has been challenged by the observation of intersubjectivity scholars that the newborn is an active initiator of dialogical interaction from the very beginning of life (Bråten & Treaverthen, 2007; Stern, 2004; Trevarthen, 2001). The newborn has been found to have an inherited sympathetic capacity to actively participate in a dialogical relationship by attuning to the other by rhythmically synchronizing his or her movements with those of the adult. This "jazz-like" rhythmicity—Colwyn Trevarthen's expression—occurs in movement, vocalization, and later speech. Rhythmic attunement to others forms the basis of the human mind (Gallagher, 2011; Trevarthen, 2001). We communicate through our movements and by responding to the movements of others, and we become human in relation to others by synchronizing these movements musically and rhythmically. Primary sympathetic intersubjective interaction carries the newborn for about the first 6 months of life and then in the stage of secondary intersubjectivity the child learns to read the mind of the other in active interaction with itself. Reading the mind of the other does not mean that the child understands the mind of the adult as an external, independent phenomenon, but in the shared common encounter and experience of interpersonal relationships (Gallagher, 2011). The child "reads the other's mind" in relationship to them here and now.

When we come into the world, we are equipped with two fundamental capacities. We learn to breathe, which is essential for oxygen and vital functions. If we do not learn to breathe, we will die. In the same way, we learn to dialogue, to initiate, and to respond. If we do not learn to dialogue, we will die. Bakhtin said that when dialogue ends, everything ends. Beyond that is death. So, dialogue is a basic form of life, like breathing. We all need dialogue because without it we cannot live. There is no point in asking what is the indication for dialogue, and whether there are any contraindications to it. Dialogue is always and, in all cases, needed, all our clients can benefit from it. Of course, the form of dialogue will vary according to the specific circumstances of each situation. The very essence of dialogue also means that the very act of dialogue is a healing experience in itself because, in a dialogical relationship, the person becomes himself. It also means that even a small baby becomes the author of her own growth through a dialogical relationship. While traditionally we think of parents as raising their children, through an understanding of intersubjectivity the child is no longer the object of upbringing, but an active agent in her own growth. In the same way, when an adult encounters a problem and needs help, he/she is no longer the object of care but the active agent of his own care. It is then possible to mobilize many more resources to build a future.

Research on intersubjectivity has focused on the experience of one child or the interaction between two people—an adult and a child. This is understandable in terms of constructing challenging research designs, as it is a very multidimensional phenomenon. But life is not essentially a two-centered affair; from the very beginning, a baby's life is constructed from multiple relational experiences, which may also be actively present at the same time. For example, the psychoanalyst Reis (2010) criticizes psychoanalysis for overemphasizing bilateral intersubjectivity. Fivaz-Depeursinge and Corboz-Warnery (1999) argued that a very crucial step in child development takes place from a bilateral to a trilateral relationship situation, where the child acts with two adults simultaneously. In such a situation, the participant becomes attuned first and foremost to the other people involved in the situation before attuning to the task to be performed. The simultaneous experiences of multiple relationships are stored in the child's body memory and, when given verbal expression, become voices of the mind that are activated in each interaction. It is important to stress that the voices of the mind are not so much a metaphor for multiple simultaneous meanings of things but are concrete interpersonal experiences of bodily memory. They are not stored in body memory as complete narratives but are stored in each sensory area in a manner specific to that sense, and voices are always combined into an experience in an interpersonal situation that in some ways resembles the original experiences (Damasio, 1999).

The polyphony of the human mind—living in many voices—is expressed in this way. In one therapy situation, the client was asked to write a letter to his deceased father. He wrote a very vivid letter with metaphors that illustrated his experience. When he was asked to write a reply to himself in his father's voice, the language of the letter was very different, reduced, and concrete. When the therapists pointed out the difference in the language of the two letters, he said that he himself immediately noticed the difference. He had not done it deliberately, but the language just took shape on its own. When he wrote in his father's voice, the memory of his father in his body shaped his sensorimotor activity. The father's voice lives in the body's memory and directly influences the body's functions.

The human brain is shaped by embodied experiences of this kind in dialogical relationships with other people (Tomasello et al., 2005). The development of the surface layer of the cerebral cortex is closely related to the heightened sociality of the human mind, which includes the ability to cooperate, the intersubjective ability to understand the mind of others, and culture. These features of brain activity occur by mobilizing primarily the right hemisphere regions of the brain, in the area of implicit knowledge in synchrony with interpersonal relationships (Porges, 2011; Quillman, 2012; Schore, 2009). Implicit knowledge is experience that is bound up with emotional experience, which may not have a clear explicit account of its experience. That is precisely what William James was talking about when he sought to define human experience as sensations without a verbal explicit description.

The Human Mind as an Embodied Relational Experience

The human mind can be seen as a process that takes two forms in human relationships. First, it takes place in the relationship of present interaction. All things experienced take on meaning in the present moment in the presence of these people. Secondly, the human mind is constructed from all the relational experiences in the body's memory, which are shaped into the voices of life according to the theme of each interaction. They form the inner voices of mind. Both dimensions are present in all interactional situations, whereby the relational mind (Gregory Bateson's concept, 1972) is realized as a process of synchronization of all participants with one another. The human mind is active in the synchronization of the participants, as much in the autonomic nervous system, as in the central nervous system as much as in the spoken language. On the other hand, it is activated by the activation of internal voices, for example, in response to some memories or in the processing of traumatic bodily experiences. In the process of memory of traumatic bodily experiences, the emphasis is mostly on implicit experiences, so that their meaning emerges in the process of responding as a unique experience for each participant. The autonomic nervous system plays a very special role here, since both the arousal of the sympathetic nervous system and the activity of the parasympathetic nervous system from arousal to recovery occur mainly outside the conscious will, before it. William James and Maurice Merleau-Ponty (1962) saw the human mind as a relational process, manifesting itself in time rather than place. The human mind is not primarily an invisible property operating inside the head. As I noted earlier, for William James, the metaphor that best describes the human mind is flow, rather than fixed categories. Flow is an ever-moving process in which we experience things such as sensations and in which we are constantly influencing each other's emotional sensations.

Participatory Sensemaking: Participatory Reasoning

Professors Thomas Fuchs and Hanne de Jaegher (De Jaegher, 2019; Fuchs & De Jaegher, 2009; Fuchs Koch, 2014) from Heidelberg provided an interesting insight into the role of intersubjectivity in understanding social cognition (perception, thinking, and reasoning). They described the new sociality of phenomenology in the era of intersubjectivity and intercorrelativity. For them too, sociality and social cognition is an embodied activity. They criticized the tendency of traditional brain research to explain cognition only in terms of the brain's ability to create a picture of the phenomenon being cognized. Many brain scientists may also be interested in intersubjectivity, but for them, intersubjectivity is more a background to thinking, reasoning, and perception, not an organic part of cognition. For example, according to Fuchs and DeJaegher, mirror cell research has often been interested in the processes taking place in the observer's mirror neurons rather than describing the whole reciprocal event. However, mirror neuron function cannot be understood without its connection to a meaningful interaction situation.

They use the term "enactive" to describe an intersubjective process in which an actor always responds to the initiatives of another person present. These responses, in turn, initiate the responses of others, which become initiatives, and so on, indefinitely. For them, intersubjectivity is both an interactive and an individual phenomenon. It is always linked to the body's dynamic relationship with its environment. The origins and aspirations of action are not hidden but are always manifested in action and thus readable by the participants in situations. These starting points and aspirations are openly influenced and are not fixed. The participants in the interaction are constantly influencing each other, and the interaction itself becomes an active subject. Social consciousness is constructed through embodied interaction.

In this interaction, the parties are synchronized with each other, but it is important to understand that this synchronization is never perfect. The imperfection of synchronization is essential in an evolution that is constantly in flux because it gives rise to new interest and a new drive to take interactive initiatives to understand the other's point of view. Thus, misunderstandings and irritations, for example, are essential to social interaction and to the pursuit of synchronization.

Their concept differs from the traditional description of social cognition, which is thought to create internal representations and images of external reality. In their description, the essential is built on the interaction between the participants, where all the efforts and impulses to move forward are generated. The outputs of interaction are often surprising and cannot be predicted. On the other hand, everything happens in a culturally specific context and under specific conditions, which create the framework for interaction in this particular cultural situation, where not all is possible.

Interestingly, De Jaegher (2019) describes knowing as an experience of love. The knower and the object of knowing can no longer be separated but are as closely linked as in a love relationship.

Intersubjectivity of Dialogical Therapy Conversations

What does this mean for therapeutic conversations? We can bear in mind the meeting between family and caring network described in Chap. 2 and its powerful emotional experiences. Is it sufficient, then, to have a shared, dialogical experience without a specific therapeutic intervention in which the clients and therapists in the conversation create meaning for the stories told?

In his dialogical worldview, Bakhtin saw getting a response as the most important human experience. Not having a response is, according to him, the most terrible human experience. For him, the most important thing is that we find ourselves in our expressions if we can find an answer to them. Here, the answer is not understood as a verbal explanation of how what is said should be understood, but as the experience of being recognized and accepted. "I see myself in your eyes," he might have said.

When I see myself in the eyes of another, the response is a non-verbal, immediate, and unmediated experience.

Elsewhere, psychiatrists Tom Andersen and Daniel Stern also provide an important contribution to the description of the therapeutic situation. Stern described this new revolutionary view of man as having fundamentally changed his psychotherapy. No longer are the therapist's interpretations aimed at explaining the client's narrative, but at encouraging the client's experience in the here and now. He says they have given up guiding the client in any way. In the therapy session, the client's narrative is followed and responded to in the here and now.

In the last years of his life, Andersen (2007) became interested in a third kind of reality, which takes the form of bodily experiences, mostly without words, in the here and now. He described this with the words not—and not. We might say that this experience is neither here nor there, but I know that something is happening. This is what he considered most important. Narrative therapy, which emphasizes the centrality of language, stresses the importance of having several different accounts of the same thing. This is what Andersen named as being in the both—and in reality. Both what you say and what I say are equally valuable in our joint efforts to understand difficult things. Tom Andersen saw this as an important step towards a conversation that respects all experiences. But beyond this, for him, it is primary and even more important to capture something of the experience that occurs before it is put into words. This experience is always created in the moment. Both Stern and Andersen thus seem to emphasize that the (embodied) experience that emerges in the discourse takes precedence over the content of what is spoken. In my own therapy work, this is an increasingly important principle. It is not so important that we discuss exactly the right things because while speaking about many things, we can share something of that embodied experience for which there are not yet words. In fact, all roads (of conversation) can lead to Rome!

This was well illustrated in the therapy meeting in Chap. 2. We followed up closely on the issues raised by family members. We did not make any corrective suggestions by saying, for example, that it would be important to talk about this or that topic as well. Both in this discussion and in previous discussions, the family members had, as Natalia said, developed a new experience of each other and of their suffering.

Natalia: Well…. I'm a super fan of this way of working, so it works for me. If you ask me how to improve it, I think we already have everything! Today, listening to my mom, I felt staggered because my mom is very reserved, she doesn't usually talk about her feelings. And now to see her bring all these things here with great understanding… it makes me feel even more… When I try… if my sister wants to, because therapy doesn't work, if the person doesn't want to, she can also bring her own issues as a person, as a mother, and everything else. So, I really like this model and how our therapists work. It works for me!

It's as if we're always in two meetings at the same time. We are in a verbal meeting where we discuss the important issues raised by clients. And at the same time, we are always in a meeting right here and now, sharing a new shared experience. This new shared experience produces new words and new language for experiences that have not yet been put into words. When the anxiety and pain that lives in our bodily experience begins to be shared, there is room for new ideas and new ways of dealing with our own pain, as Natalia said.

In family therapy, this new dimension has increased the possibilities for dealing with difficult crises. But family therapy—and psychotherapy in general—has in the past focused most of its attention on spoken language. How then has the shift from the primacy of spoken language to an emphasis on a shared experience of sharing taken place? This is the subject of the next chapter.

References

Andersen, T. (2007). Human participating: Human 'being' is the step for human 'becoming' in the next step. In H. Anderson & D. Gehart (Eds.), *Collaborative therapy: Relationships and conversations that make a difference* (pp. 81–94). Routledge/Taylor & Francis.

Bateson, G. (1972). *Steps to an ecology of mind: A revolutionary approach to man's understanding of himself.* Random House.

Bråten, S., & Treaverthen, C. (2007). From infant intersubjectivity and participant movements to stimulation and conversation in cultural common sense. In S. Bråten (Ed.), *On being moved: From mirror neurons to empathy* (pp. 21–34). John Benjamin.

Damasio, A. (1999). *The feeling of what happens.* Mariner Books.

De Jaegher, H. (2019). Loving and knowing. Reflections for an engaged epistemology. *Phenomenology and the Cognitive Sciences.* https://doi.org/10.1007/s11097-019-09634-5

Fivaz-Depeursinge, E., & Corboz-Warnery, A. (1999). *The primary triangle. A developmental systems view of mothers, fathers and infants.* Basic Books.

Fuchs, T., & De Jaegher, H. (2009). Enactive intersubjectivity: Participatory sense-making and mutual incorporation. *Phenomenological Cognitive Sciences, 465–486.* https://doi.org/10.1007/s11097-009-9136-4

Fuchs, T., & Koch, S. (2014). Embodied affectivity: On moving and being moved. *Frontiers in Psychology, 5.* https://doi.org/10.3389/fpsyg.2014.00508

Gallagher, S. (2011). In defence of phenomenological approaches to social cognition: Intersecting with the critics. *The Review of Philosophy and Psychology.* https://doi.org/10.1007/s13164-011-0080-1

Hughes, D. (2015). *Attachment-focused family therapy - Interactive developmental psychotherapy.*

Mahler, S., Pine, M. M., & Bergman, A. (1973). *The psychological birth of the human infant.* Basic Books.

Merleau-Ponty, M. (1962). *Phenomenology of perception* (C. Smith, Trans.). Routledge and Kegan Paul.

Porges, S. (2011). *The polyvagal theory: Neurophysiological foundations of emotions, attachment, communication, self-regulation.* Norton.

Quillman, T. (2012). Neuroscience and therapist self-disclosure: Deepening right brain to right brain communication between therapist and patient. *Clinical Social Work Journal, 40,* 1–9.

Reis, B. (2010). A human family: Commentary on paper by Elisabeth Fivaz-Depeursinge, Chloe Lavanchy-Scaiola, and Nicolas Favez. *Psychoanalytic Dialogues, 20,* 151–157.

Schore, A. (2009). Right brain affect regulation: An essential mechanism of development, trauma, dissociation, and psychotherapy. In D. Fosha & D. Siegel (Eds.), *The healing power of emotion: Affective neuroscience, development & clinical practice* (pp. 112–144). Norton.

Sheet-Johnstone, M. (2010). *The corporeal turn. An interdisciplinary reader.* Imprint Academic.

Shotter, J. (2011). *Getting it: Withness-thinking and the dialogical in practice.* Hampton Press.

Siegel, D. (2010). *Mindsight. The science of change*. Basam Books.
Stern, D. (2004). *The present moment in psychotherapy and everyday life*. Norton.
Tomasello, M., Carpenter, M., Call, J., Behne, T., & Moll, H. (2005). Understanding and sharing intentions: The origins of cultural cognition. *Behavioral and Brain Sciences, 28*, 675–691.
Trevarthen, C. (2001). Intrinsic motives for companionship in understanding: Their origin, development, and significance for infant mental health. *Infant Mental Health Journal, 23*, 95–131.
Vygotsky, L. (1930). The functions of sign in the development of higher mental processes. In R. Wieber & D. Robinson (Eds.) (2004). The essential Vygotsky (p. 543). Luwer Academic.
Vygotsky, L. (1935/1982). *Thought and language*. MIT Press.

Chapter 5
The Evolution of Family Therapy from Systemic to Embodied Sharing

In the previous chapters, we have shared how our view of human being has changed due to dialogue practice and the importance of this change in our view of humanity in order to better help those who need help. The focus is on family therapy. Open Dialogue has evolved as a family therapy practice so that the aim is no longer to change the family system, but to create a shared experience in which a new language for managing the most difficult experiences emerges. Families are not the objects of treatment but indispensable partners. Born in the tradition of need-adapted care and a key event in Open Dialogue, the therapy meeting is not really family therapy, but it can be seen applying ideas of family therapy. My thesis is that the shift from systemic family therapy to a dialogical shared experience has been instrumental in improving treatment outcomes in the most difficult crises.

On Family Systems

In family therapy, meetings involve several people—both family members and clinicians—who work together in harmony to create a healing partnership. It is a multi-actor conversation. To understand the options for multiagency dialogues, in this chapter, I will explore the change that has taken place in family therapy. It is worth remembering that in family therapy, the emergence of the human mind takes place in multiple relationships.

Without the change in family therapy, dialogical therapy meetings could not have become as effective in helping families—and those in the center of concern—as they have. Because we work as therapists in an interpersonal network, and because we constantly seek to match our practice to the people present, there is a synchronicity between participants in all family therapy. Therapy with families can generally be called systemic therapy because the activity takes place within the family system. But the term systemic family therapy is also closely related to one family therapy

J. Seikkula, *Why Dialogue Does Cure*,
https://doi.org/10.1007/978-3-031-91294-8_5

method, in relation to which the dialogical work described in this book is in many ways different.

When I started working as a psychologist in the late 1970s and later moved to Tornio Keropudas Hospital in the early 1980s, I became increasingly interested in the involvement of families in a patient's crisis and recovery, and I applied for training in family therapy in 1983–1986. I was very happy with that training, because even then, through that training, I came to understand more about the human being as a relational being, always functioning in interpersonal relationships. However, family therapy did not completely break away from pathology-centered thinking, which I did not understand at that time.

We arranged for family therapy teams to treat families in family therapy if we thought the family had some problems of interaction or other in some other domain of life. According to a systemic approach (Minuchin, 1974; Selvini-Palazzoli et al., 1978), problems and symptoms—for example, psychosis, depression, or eating disorders—were seen as a function of the family system. When the functioning of the family system was threatened, the role of psychological symptoms was to restore the homeostasis of the family system and to ensure the functioning of the family. This description of psychological symptoms was very radical and challenged traditional individual- and pathology-centered thinking, which saw symptoms as signs of illness and needed to be eliminated as quickly as possible. However, systemic thinking focuses primarily on the functioning of the whole family rather than the individual. A symptom can also, unexpectedly, have a positive meaning. In a family therapy discussion, this phenomenon is easily observed. When we ask a family how the illness of a family member—for example, the son of the family suffering from psychosis—has affected the relationship between the father and mother, the most frequent answer is that it has brought them closer together and has put more emphasis on family cohesion. From such a response, the systemic family therapist concluded that the function of the illness of the family son with psychosis was to increase family cohesion. In systemic family therapy, the key task is to find and influence the rules that govern the functioning of the family system.

From Systems to Language Descriptions and Narratives

The systemic view was also criticized in the 1980s. In his analysis of various shifts in psychotherapy research, Cromby (2012) referred to this new development—emerging from the critique of systemic family therapy—as the "linguistic turn". First, solution-focused therapists began to pay attention to the fact that in the family, solutions—or attempts at solutions—become problems in such a way that they begin to create a new system of action. Thus, they began to pay attention to the fact that talking about the problem in a different way changes the system. Instead of therapists and clients trying to figure out what caused the problem, it was more important to talk about what solutions to the problem might have already existed and how to strengthen them. From looking for the causes of the past, the orientation was clearly toward the present moment and the future.

Similarly, the pioneers of narrative therapy, Michael White and David Epston, began to pay attention to the power of problem-saturated narratives in life. The focus was on the narratives that each individual had formed about life in general and the problematic situation in particular. They based their ideas on descriptions by many sociologists and philosophers of how narratives dominate life. The descriptions of the French sociologist Michael Foucault, for example, were very important for understanding the power that dominant narratives have in life. When problems take over narratives, they become thin narratives, carried by only one thread—the problem. The goal of therapy becomes to thicken the thin narratives by, for example, encouraging therapy participants to reflect on the multiple meanings of the same issue. Richer and more complex narratives emerge from hearing the voices of all family members simultaneously, rather than seeking the truth of one family system.

The most obvious sign of the new turn was Harry Goolishian and Harlene Anderson's article Human systems and linguistic systems (Anderson & Goolishian, 1988) where they stated that systems do not create problems, but problems create systems. According to them, a family problem gives rise to a specific way of talking and acting in the family that eventually dominates the whole system. They were the first to describe family therapy as a dialogical process. According to them, the aim is not to solve problems, but to dis-solve them in a dialogue that creates new meanings. The aim of the therapeutic work is to create a dialogue so that the voices of all the participants in the discussion are heard, so that their understanding can be transformed.

Therapy trends that emphasize the centrality of language are closely related to social constructionism. The most significant breakthrough in understanding social constructionism was made by Berger and Luckmann (1994) in their 1966 book. They argued that people interact to create meanings about each other and in the process these meanings begin to determine each other's actions, forming different roles. These roles gradually become institutionalized, creating a socially constructed reality. Social interaction, they argue, determines both our social status and the reality of our lives. Language is, of course, very central to the construction of the institutions that define our social lives. Kenneth Gergen and John Shotter, in close collaboration with family therapists, created a description of social reality. Social constructionism focuses on the description of reality; in family therapy, for example, this means that the aim of therapy is to create a kind of discourse in which different people are encouraged to share their own description of a phenomenon they perceive as a problem. If the speaker is heard, this increases the complexity and relationality of the understanding of the problem. In such a polyphonic discussion, the problem definition gradually begins to unravel.

The approach has its merits. It provides a good starting point for dealing with the most difficult crises. The knowledge we need is always built up in each unique encounter—it is contextual. Experiences that seem difficult begin to take on new meaning in the here and now, as happened in the therapy meeting in Chap. 2. Reality is not an object of observation independent of us and outside of us, but is constantly being created by our own perceptions and descriptions. Reality is not so much seen as constructed by each individual in his or her own mind, but we create our reality between the participants in each situation, in relationship.

In the early 1990s, the dialogical approach in family therapy and psychiatry began to develop as part of these methods that emphasize the centrality of language. In psychiatric care in Western Lapland, we began to call this new way of working Open Dialogue. The dialogical orientation emphasizes more than the narrative approach the importance of each moment for the emergence of new meanings. People talk about events in their lives, but what matters most is the response these stories get in the here and now. The therapist's task is to respond to clients' expressions in a way that makes them feel heard. The therapist's role changes so that the clients guide the therapeutic work and the therapists, through their responses, synchronize their own actions with the clients' expressions, so that all participants in the dialogue are attuned to each other in both the content of what is said and the way it is said.

From Linguistic Descriptions to Embodied Participation in Dialogue

But this is not only the result of linguistic descriptions. It always involves the complete experience of the participants in the conversation, including bodily sensations. It is not just a question of describing reality and the problem it poses, but of those who describe reality becoming part of this event—as bodily present and constantly experiencing it—and in this way affecting and changing the reality, in which they participate. As the discussion progresses, the experience also changes. The participants in the discussion experience everything that is said in their immediate emotional sensations and thoughts. In addition to this, they experience each other as being present and affecting all the time. When I am interacting, I am always responding to what I am experiencing under the influence of another person, and, again, my bodily presence affects the others present. It may sound complicated, but in fact, it is self-evident. For example, if I am in the presence of an angry speaker, my own irritation rises—which in turn becomes part of my emotional experience and the meaning that arises from it.

The overemphasis on the linguistic construction of reality also gradually began to be criticized. Already in the early 1990s, John Shotter—one of the scholars of social constructionism—spoke of human as embodied being (Shotter, 1993). Later, he pointed out that the problem with social constructionism is that it is not radical enough, because the construction of reality as linguistic descriptions does not take into account the reality's descriptors as concrete participants in situations. We are present in every event with our own bodies, and this bodily participation inevitably becomes part of the reality we create in our linguistic representations. For example, simply moving from one corner of a room to the center of the room changes our perception of space in a fundamental way.

The perspective of embodied participation in situations adds a whole new dimension to the understanding of linguistically constructed reality. Some psychotherapists had long before emphasized the importance of embodiment in therapeutic situations. Andersen (1991, 2007, 2022), together with colleagues, developed the concept of reflective processes. Andersen's focus is on how the client is breathing and how the therapist's questions must be sufficiently different from the client's way of thinking to evoke a new experience. According to Andersen, this is reflected in a change in breathing when inhaling. However, the therapist's questions and comments cannot be too different, because then it is easy for the client's breathing to become blocked, and new learning does not take place. If, on the other hand, the therapist's comments and questions are too ordinary in relation to the client's experience, they will have no effect on the change in breathing and will not open up curiosity for new perspectives. In Andersen's description, bodily involvement through breathing is directly related to the progression of the therapeutic dialogue.

According to Mikhail Bakhtin, dialogue is itself an embodied activity. Bakhtin made two extremely important points: (1) we participate in dialogue with all our actions and with our whole body, not only by speaking. Of course, speech is also a bodily activity. (2) Bodily participation takes place throughout life, from the first inhalation to the last exhalation. Thus, embodiment is an integral part of dialogicity. It is not just a question of a social reality created in narratives, as in narrative therapy, but of active bodily participation in the reality we describe all the time.

Psychotherapy has traditionally been understood as the construction of meaning in verbal language. The Western concept of man has been dominated by the dualistic view of man originally described by Rene Descartes in 1637 (Descartes, 2001). According to this view, body and soul, feeling and reason can be separated. In the field of psychotherapy, the dualistic conception of man is still much alive. The central function of psychotherapy is thought to be the life experiences narrated in the therapeutic conversation and the meanings given to them in the therapist's responses. This type of thinking builds up many models of, for example, the construction of the human psyche according to specific categories. The best known of these is the psychoanalytic view of the human being, the structure of the ego and of the self. A therapeutic description based on language and the centrality of the meanings given to the narrative remains a dualistic view of the human being, since only verbal explanations are central to it.

According to Cromby, the linguistic turn was followed by an "affective turn." In describing psychotherapy, several authors have explored this, including Damasio and Carvalho (2013), Schore (2009) and Stern (2004). The focus is not on the narratives told in words, but on how the emotional awakening of the participants in the interaction takes place as they process their life experiences here and now. William James described this as sensation. In the flow of life, we sense similarities and dissimilarities in our bodies, most of which do not take any precise shape, but are really sensory-like glimmers of something. These glimpses and sensations are not yet feelings. Usually in psychotherapy, when talking about emotions, we refer to the ability of clients to put into words a description of an emotion they are feeling—for example, sadness or anxiety—about an insult they have experienced. Such emotions are in fact thoughts that already involve a great deal of rational reasoning (Damasio, 1999). It therefore occurs after the sensory processing of emotions. Attention to affective arousal tends to catch the experience at the moment of its occurrence before it is put into words. This happens, for example, when the speaker is moved in mid-sentence by something he or she has said. The sensation occurs alongside or before the words and describes a situation in which someone does not yet have a narrative to describe. Mental symptoms are an example of sensations that are not yet verbalized by the body. In anxiety, the heart starts beating faster; in depression, there is a change in blood pressure; in psychotic hallucination, there is a cortical vibration or pre-movement of the vocal cords. These sensations are at the heart of dialogical family therapy and Open Dialogues.

The Elements of Synchronization

Family therapy is a multi-actor activity where everyone takes each other into account. Consideration of the other is not only in speech, but in all activities. It is a matter of synchronizing bodily functions, of adjusting them to each other. Clients with each other, therapists with each other, and clients and therapists synchronize in many ways. Figure 5.1 summarizes the aspects of synchronization in couples' therapy.

In therapy, we adapt to each other first of all in the spoken language. There are two dimensions to spoken language: (1) what we talk about (the content of speech) and (2) how we talk (the prosody of speech), both of which are at least partly the volitional activity of the participant in the conversation, although the prosodic dimensions of speech in particular (volume, pitch, and pauses) also contain many elements that we do not consciously control.

The two parts of the autonomic nervous system (ANS) respond autonomically, not voluntarily. Any stimulus we receive triggers the sympathetic nervous system (SNS) to respond and stimulates us into action. It helps us, for example, to defend ourselves or to develop an emotion. The parasympathetic nervous system (PNS), on the other hand, returns us to action from a state of arousal. It is through the autonomic nervous system that we are most directly connected to the reality around us. As part of the environment, the people involved in each conversation, through their actions and sensations, are constantly influencing and being influenced by each other.

Body movements and postures are part of our emotional regulation and communication. They are synchronized into the conversation mostly outside of our voluntary control, but some of our body movements can also be chosen in the flow of the conversation. Facial movements are apparently the most sensitive part of human communication. This is particularly related to smiling as part of an initiative on the part of another and responding to the initiative of another. Similarly, gaze alignment

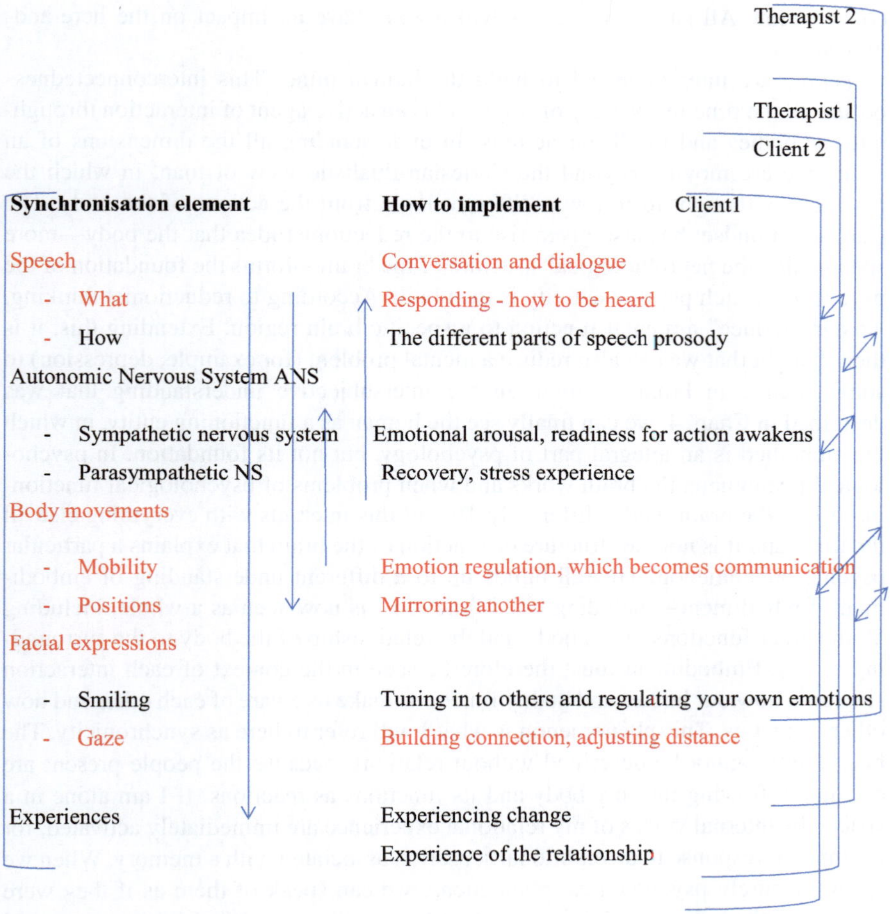

Fig. 5.1 Factors of internal and intersubjective synchronization. Example of a couple therapy situation between two therapists and a couple. In the figure, the red color indicates that this action is volitional and the black color indicates that the action is outside volitional control

is an essential part of synchronization. For example, when agitated or frightened, we may look at the lower part of the other's face rather than directly into their eyes.

The last part of the synchronicity presented here is our experience of the conversation. These experiences orient our actions already in this conversation and especially in the following ones. Our experiences guide us to analyze them in our minds and to take this into account, for example, in our next comments in the conversation. The same always happens in the next discussion, where we orient ourselves on the previous discussion. I try to make my points more clearly, I try to argue even more comprehensively, I try to correct a factual error that occurred in the previous conversation, I try to regulate my emotional experience better than I did in yesterday's conversation. All such experiences will always have an impact on the here-and-now debate.

People are interconnected to build the human mind. This interconnectedness occurs all the time in a variety of ways and is an active agent of interaction throughout our bodies and in all our actions. In understanding all the dimensions of an event, we are moving beyond the Cartesian dualistic view of man, in which the psyche was thought to follow a different logic from the actions of the body. The Cartesian mindset has also given rise to the reductionist idea that the body—more specifically, the neurobiological structure of the brain—forms the foundation of the psyche, on which psychic activity is then built. According to reductionist thinking, we can "reduce" a mental function to a specific brain region. Extending this, it is then thought that we can also reduce a mental problem (for example, depression) to some change in brain function. In the intersubjective understanding that was described in Chap. 4, we can finally see the human as a functioning entity, in which the embodied is an integral part of psychology, but not its foundation. In psychological phenomena the brain works and when problems of psychological functioning occur, the brain works differently. But all this interacts with everything else all the time, and it is not the structure or function of the brain that explains a particular psychic phenomenon. This all builds up to a different understanding of embodiment. Embodiment—including brain function—is now seen as a whole, including all the other functions of the body and the relationship of the body to the surrounding reality. Embodiment must therefore be seen in the context of each interaction situation, how our bodies and bodily functions make us aware of each other and how others affect us. This phenomenon is what I will refer to here as synchronicity. The bodily self cannot be described without relations, because the people present are constantly flowing into my body and its functions as reactions. If I am alone in a space, the internal voices of my relational experience are immediately activated, for example in response to an emotional sensation associated with a memory. When we speak of purely psychological phenomena, we can speak of them as if they were intrinsic to the individual. We can speak of personality traits ("he is a temperamental person" or "he is selfish") or of the unconscious as if they were phenomena within the person without a relationship to the outside world, but when we move to a comprehensive integrated description, taking into account the embodiment of the individual, this is no longer possible.

The embodiment perspective also helps to define cognition—the reasoning that takes place in thinking—more broadly. Cognition has tended to be seen as taking place in the brain, for example by generating various metaphors so that computer models of brain activity can be created to predict human behavior. Tschacher and Bergomi (2011) criticize this view, arguing that the embodiment view goes beyond a neurobiological model of cognition. We now understand that all bodily functions—such as facial expressions, movements, speech prosody, gestures, and body postures—affect the human mind and are areas of influence of the human mind. Thus, the study of embodiment cannot be limited to neurobiological methods and the study of the functioning of the human brain, but must include the study of human activity in all its diversity. Neurobiological research has indeed made significant advances in our understanding of the human mind, but the human mind cannot be understood by looking only at brain function.

The Study of Rhythmic Synchrony in Psychotherapy

Embodiment has also gained ground in psychotherapy research. In his study, Quillman (2012) followed individual psychotherapy as a communication between the right hemispheres of the brain of two people. In the study, the therapists actively expressed their own emotional, implicit experiences. Lapides (2011) carried out a similar activity in couples therapy by observing the stimulation of clients' sympathetic nervous systems. When the study tracked what the clients' autonomic nervous system primarily responded to in the therapist's intervention, it was found that it did not respond mainly to the content of the therapist's speech. Therapy clients responded primarily to the prosody of the therapist's speech—i.e., changes in rhythm, pitch and volume of speech—and to the therapist's body postures, gestures, and facial expressions. One can well assume that the same happens in any kind of dialogue, for example between friends, in a family, or at a therapy meeting. It is how we speak that is more important than the content of our speech.

In couples therapy, Atkinson (2013), Fishbane (2011), Gottman (2011), Johnson (2013) and Solomon and Tatkin (2011) considered embodiment as part of the interaction in the therapy situation. Johnson and Solomon & Tatkin did so in the context of attachment theory, and Atkinson in relation to mindfulness. Fishbane provides neurobiological information in helping the couple both to control their own emotional regulation and, at the same time, to become more compassionate to their spouse's emotions. Patterson and Vakili (2014) have sought to provide family therapists with information on how to use the new neuroscience research in their therapeutic practice. John Gottman has developed a way of working to consider emotional distortion in the therapy situation. He and his research team have published studies on the role of emotions in relationship conflict, divorce, and intimate partner violence (Driver & Gottman, 2004; Gottman & Levenson, 2000; Jacobson et al., 1996). By observing spouses' reactions under specific research conditions (i.e. not in the therapy situation itself), they found that emotional distortion in the autonomic nervous system of the male spouse was one of six predictors of divorce.

The above studies have examined the physical responses of clients. It is not yet synchronization because it does not take therapists into account. Once the therapist(s) are accounted for in the studies, we understand more about intersynchrony in psychotherapy. Ramseyer and Tschacher (2011) found a strong relationship between the amount of synchrony between therapist and client body movements and perceived collaborative alliance. The more body movement synchrony occurred, the better both the therapist and the client perceived the working alliance, which in turn seemed to predict better therapeutic outcome. Fuchs and Koch (2014) found a link between body movements and perceived emotions and relational states, and how these manifest in the interactional situation of psychotherapy. In a study published with Avdi et al. (2015), we found that bodily synchrony between therapist and client was at its highest during deviations in the therapeutic alliance (e.g. ruptures, misunderstanding), that is, when problems were experienced in the therapeutic working alliance. Bänninger-Huber and Widmer (1999) investigated recurrent emotional experiences in the therapeutic relationship, with particular reference to guilt. They developed a specific research method, the Facial Action Coding System (FACS), based on Ekman and Friesen's (1978) original observation that six basic emotions can be detected by facial muscle movements. In particular, Bänninger-Huber and Widmer investigated prototypical affective microsequences (PAMs), which are expressed primarily in non-linguistically repetitive smiles and chuckles that regulate the therapeutic relationship between client and therapist.

Darwiche et al. (2008) found reciprocal moments of smiling to be a key aspect of the therapist–client triad in couples therapy to express emotional experience and regulate the mutual relationship. Using their MSE (Mutual Smiling Episode) Coding System (MSE-CS) methodology, they further identified forms of support, mutual bonding, sharing suffering, restorative experience, and challenge in regulating the therapist–client relationship. The more frequently these small events were observed, the better the therapeutic alliance was perceived to be. Benecke et al. (2005) also found an association between simultaneous smiling and perceived relationship satisfaction.

There have also been some interesting observations on the stimulation of the autonomic nervous system of therapists. Kleinbub et al. (2012) compared the sympathetic nervous system activation of a trained psychotherapist, a newly qualified psychologist, and a layperson in a mock client situation. The layperson's electrodermal activity—measured via skin electrical conductivity—was not significantly related to the client's response. The newly qualified psychologist had a negative correlation with client's nervous system arousal. In contrast, a trained psychotherapist had a positive correlation with client's sympathetic nervous system arousal. Thus, the therapist and the client experienced things in the same way in their autonomic nervous systems, especially the sympathetic nervous system. The researchers interpreted this to mean that, during therapy training, the therapist's sympathetic nervous system is slowed down to the extent that cognitive reasoning becomes possible at the same time as intense emotional experiences. According to Decety et al. (2007), empathic experience implies experiencing the same emotion as another and, in addition, the possibility of cognitive analysis and regulation of one's own emotion. In Chap. 8, I will delve into this topic by considering the role of increased reflexivity in therapeutic change.

The Stages of Development Are Not Categorical

I hope you didn't get tired of reading those many references to different studies. Unfortunately, we do not yet have a complete overview of how therapists and clients synchronize with each other and to each other. So, the only way to approach this important question is to report individual research findings. However, some coherent plot is beginning to emerge from them. They add a very relevant dimension to the description of family therapy. Here, I have precisely chosen those studies that help to understand the human embodied and relational mind.

The development of family therapy already has quite a long history. The systemic, linguistic, and embodied stages of family therapy are neither categorical nor mutually exclusive. The experience of different working methods enriches family therapy all the time. Although we are beginning to consider interaction as a whole, including its embodied dimension, we can still understand family therapy from a systemic point of view. Nor does the embodied perspective exclude the narrative aspect of family therapy and the importance of listening to the different experiences of family members. All these elements are also present in the dialogical encounter, even if we abandon interventions that seek to change the family. On this basis, we built our own research at the University of Jyväskylä to understand the human mind in and as constructed by relationships. It will be described in the next chapter.

References

Andersen, T. (1991). *The reflecting team*. Norton.

Andersen, T. (2007). Human participating: Human 'being' is the step for human 'becoming' in the next step. In H. Anderson & D. Gehart (Eds.), *Collaborative therapy: Relationships and conversations that make a difference* (pp. 81–94). Routledge/Taylor & Francis.

Andersen, T. (2022). *Wandering and turning points. A book about touch, involvement in psychiatry and other peace work. Helsinki.*

Anderson, H., & Goolishian, H. (1988). Human systems as linguistic systems: Preliminary and evolving ideas about the implications for clinical theory. *Family Process, 27*, 371–393.

Atkinson, B. (2013). Mindfulness training and the cultivation of secure, satisfying couple relationships. *Couple and Family Psychology: Research and Practice, 2*(2), 73–94.

Avdi, E., Lerou, V., & Seikkula, J. (2015). Dialogical features, therapist responsiveness, and agency in a therapy for psychosis. *Journal of Constructivist Psychology, 28*(4), 329–341.

Bänninger-Huber, E., & Widmer, C. (1999). Affective relationship patterns and psychotherapeutic change. *Psychotherapy Research, 9*, 74–87.

Benecke, C., Peham, D., & Bänninger-Huber, E. (2005). Nonverbal relationship regulation in psychotherapy. *Psychotherapy Research, 15*(1–2), 81–90.

Berger, P., & Luckmann, T. (1994). *The social construction of reality: A sociological study of knowledge. Postscript: Tapio Aittola and Vesa Raiskila*. Gaudeamus.

Cromby, J. (2012). Feeling the way: Qualitative clinical research and the affective turn. *Qualitative Research in Psychology, 9*, 88–98.

Damasio, A. (1999). *The feeling of what happens*. Mariner Books.

Damasio, A., & Carvalho, G. (2013). The nature of feelings: Evolutionary and neurobiological origins. *Nature, 14*, 143–152.

Darwiche, J., de Roten, Y., Stern, D., von Roten, F. C., Corboz-Warnery, A., & Fivaz-Depeursinge, E. (2008). Mutual smiling episodes and therapeutic alliance in a therapist-couple discussion task. *Swiss Journal of Psychology, 67*(4), 231–239.

Decety, J., Jackson, P., & Brunet, E. (2007). The cognitive neuropsychology of empathy. *Empathy in Mental Illness, 2007*, 239–744.

Descartes, R. (2001). *The presentation of a method. In Works 1* (Sami Jansson, Trans.). Helsinki: Gaudeamus. (Original work published 1637).

Driver, J., & Gottman, J. (2004). Daily marital interactions and positive affect during marital conflict among newlywed couples. *Family Process, 43*, 301–314.

Ekman, P., & Friesen, W. V. (1978). *Facial action coding system: A technique for the measurement of facial movement*. Consulting Psychologists Press.

Fishbane, M. (2011). Facilitating relational empowerment in couple therapy. *Family Process, 50*, 337–352.

Fuchs, T., & Koch, S. (2014). Embodied affectivity: On moving and being moved. *Frontiers in Psychology, 5*. https://doi.org/10.3389/fpsyg.2014.00508

Gottman, J. (2011). *The science of trust: Emotional attunement for couples*. W. W. Norton & Company.

Gottman, J., & Levenson, R. (2000). The timing of divorce: Predicting when a couple will divorce over a 14-year period. *Journal of Marriage and the Family, 62*, 737–745.

Jacobson, N., Gottman, J. M., Gortner, E., Berns, S., & Shortt, J. W. (1996). Psychological factors in the longitudinal course of battering: When do the couples split up? When does the abuse decrease? *Violence Victims, 11*(4), 371–392.

Johnson, S. (2013). *Love sense. The revolutionary new science of romantic relationships*. Little, Brown and Company.

Kleinbub, J., Messina, I., Bordin, D., Voci, A., & Calvo, V. (2012). Synchronization of skin conductance levels in therapeutic dyads. *International Journal of Psychophysiology, 85*(2012), 361–430.

Lapides, F. (2011). The implicit realm in couples therapy: Improving right hemisphere affect-regulating capabilities. *Clinical Social Work Journal, 39*, 161–169.

Minuchin, S. (1974). *Families and family therapy*. Harvard University Press.

Patterson, J. E., & Vakili, S. (2014). Relationships, environment, and the brain: How emerging research is changing what we know about the impact of families on human development. *Family Process, 53*, 22–32. https://doi.org/10.1111/famp.12057

Quillman, T. (2012). Neuroscience and therapist self-disclosure: Deepening right brain to right brain communication between therapist and patient. *Clinical Social Work Journal, 40*, 1–9.

Ramseyer, F., & Tschacher, W. (2011). Nonverbal synchrony in psychotherapy: Coordinated body movement reflects relationship quality and outcome. *Journal of Consulting and Clinical Psychology, 79*(3), 284–295. https://doi.org/10.1037/a0023419

Schore, A. (2009). Right brain affect regulation: An essential mechanism of development, trauma, dissociation, and psychotherapy. In D. Fosha & D. Siegel (Eds.), *The healing power of emotion: Affective neuroscience, development & clinical practice* (pp. 112–144). Norton.

Selvini-Palazzoli, M., Boscolo, L., Cecchin, G., & Prata, G. (1978). *Paradox and Counterparadox: A new model in the therapy of the family in schizophrenic transaction*. Jason Aronson. ISBN 0876687648.

Shotter, J. (1993). *Cultural politics of every day life. Social constructionism, rhetoric and knowing of the third kind.* Open University Press.

Solomon, M., & Tatkin, S. (2011). *Love and war in intimate relationships: Connections, disconnections and mutual regulation in couple therapy*. W.W. Norton.

Stern, D. (2004). *The present moment in psychotherapy and everyday life*. Norton.

Tschacher, W., & Bergomi, C. (2011). Introduction. In W. Tschacher & C. Bergomi (Eds.), *The implications of embodiment, cognition and communication* (p. vii). Imprint Academic.

Chapter 6
Relational and Embodied Mind

The fourth part of my answer to the question of the healing power of dialogue is to understand how a dialogical approach makes it possible to consider the human being as a fully embodied being in psychotherapy. Dialogical practice draws on the knowledge that the human mind is constructed as an embodied process that enables the human being to be considered as a whole person, thereby transcending the dualistic conception of the human person. Reality emerges in each situation; it is contextual. A holistic, embodied understanding of the human mind makes psychotherapy possible to a much greater extent than before, because no longer is a special inner linguistic insight required, but the very sharing of emotional sensations is healing. Dialogical practice takes embodiment into account and thus transcends the Cartesian emphasis on the primary importance of verbal interpretations. Body and mind are connected and no longer two separate parts.

The Relational Mind Research Project

I had the wonderful opportunity to explore the meaning of embodiment in the *Human Mind* subproject (2012–2018) of the Academy of Finland-funded research program, which invited projects that would open up new understandings of the human mind in interdisciplinary research. As a condition, the research projects had to incorporate advances in modern neuroscience. For me and my colleagues, this research program came at a perfect time, when we had become interested in embodiment in psychotherapy. In this chapter, I will explain in more detail how our research project was carried out and some of the key findings. I would also like to highlight here the conduct of the research because, thanks to the creativity of the research team, we managed to create a good research design, which really allowed us to make observations about the human mind in a multi-tasking situation.

We named the project the *Relational Mind Study*. As I have already explained in previous chapters, the basic conception of the human mind is that it is realized in

J. Seikkula, *Why Dialogue Does Cure*,
https://doi.org/10.1007/978-3-031-91294-8_6

relationships in an ever-flowing stream. We borrowed the concept from social anthropologist Gregory Bateson, who was interested in life systems in general and in human interaction systems in particular. According to him, the human mind is biological and is realized in relationships. The basic premise of our research was to explore the embodiment of the human mind in a multi-actor situation. The project investigated the construction of the human mind in the interactional situation of couples therapy (Karvonen et al., 2016; Seikkula et al., 2015, 2018). Couples therapy was chosen as the subject of the study for realistic reasons, because we thought that there were no methods to study the human nervous system simultaneously if more people were involved. The study followed the whole interaction system by studying the bodily responses of the four participants (two clients and two therapists) to each other and their own emotions. The therapy sessions were recorded with a detailed facial image of each participant and a video recording of the body positions of the therapists and clients. In addition, the autonomic nervous system of both clients and therapists was measured in two sessions. Sympathetic nervous system stimulation was primarily supported by measuring skin electrical conductivity (electrodermal activity), and parasympathetic nervous system activity by measuring heart rate variability and respiration. In this way, it was possible to register how participants synchronized with each other during the couples therapy session and its emotionally stimulating discussion moments. In addition, we gained insight into how their own emotional reactions are reflected in their autonomic nervous system responses. This was investigated by showing each participant, in an individual interview, four conversation episodes perceived by the researcher as moments of change in the therapy session, simultaneously measuring both sympathetic and parasympathetic nervous system stimulation using unobserved methods.

The aim was to investigate the simultaneous influence of several factors on each other, including synchronization. In addition to synchronization, the study examined how the bodily response of each individual was related to the emotions experienced, body movements and the regulation of one's own emotional state by other means. At the same time, we looked how the other participants dealt with their own emotional states in relation to their own experiences and to each other. These were further observed both as part of conscious mind activity in spoken dialogue and in the area of autonomic nervous system stimulation outside of conscious control.

Participants in the Dialogue Also Synchronize Their Autonomic Nervous System

Dozens of scientific articles and theses have been published on the research project. Perhaps the most far-reaching finding of the project was that the sympathetic nervous system stimulation of clients and therapists does indeed synchronize with each other, creating a positive concordance between the participants (Karvonen et al., 2016). This was observed in a pairwise comparison between participants, a total of six relationship pairs in each couple's therapy session. Surprisingly, synchrony was the highest among therapists and the lowest among clients. However, synchrony between spouses increased when the couple's relationship developed positively during therapy. The study further verified that this was not a random concordance, finding that participants must indeed be in the same room for a statistically significant association to occur. Synchrony is not a random phenomenon; it is related to how individuals regulate their relationship with each other, both consciously and unconsciously. In therapy, our emotional experiences flow in parallel with those of other participants in the conversation, which is a more profound synchronization with each other than conscious empathic identification with another's situation.

Listening to a Reflective Dialogue Can Be a Stressful Experience

However, synchronization did not occur all the time or simultaneously for all four participants. Synchronicity with others manifests itself in a wide variety of ways. There are many moments in the conversation where each participant seems to react to the issue at hand and very uniquely without synchronizing their autonomic nervous responses with the others. In some situations, the sympathetic nervous system of two or three participants tuned in in synchrony after a delay of a few seconds. The same was true for the parasympathetic nervous system. In the main part of the discussion, the stress expressed by the heart rate variability is not experienced in the same way, but in some instances, the stress experiences are simultaneous and parallel (Seikkula et al., 2015). A particularly interesting recurring finding was that in the therapy conversation, the highest stress occurred while others were speaking. The other might be the spouse talking about the client and the same was true in the reflective talk between therapists, during which clients often experienced the highest levels of stress. This finding is of great importance for therapy conversations. It underlines the high emotional intensity and sensitivity of therapeutic mutual reflective talk. For clients, the stress that is generated can become a crucial learning experience, provided that the stress does not become too great. For example, if therapists use derogatory or insulting language about clients' experiences, their experience of stress may rise above the threshold of tolerance, making it impossible for them to listen to what the therapists have to say, and they begin to assert in their minds the right to their own experience. In such an emotional experience, there is no new learning or no therapeutic change.

Specifically, in couples therapy discussions related to intimate partner violence, we explore how the couple's mutual criticism and blaming of each other manifests in the stimulation of the sympathetic nervous system (Päivinen et al., 2016). In general, blaming the other person did not cause sympathetic nervous system arousal. For example, blaming the spouse for not contributing enough to joint household chores or other similar dissatisfactions in practical life. But the situation changed if the accusation was directed at the identity of the other. For example, in one conversation, the spouse accused the other of being like a child, causing a strong reaction of the sympathetic nervous system. The activation of the sympathetic nervous system is associated with the unconscious fight-or-flight response. It can be assumed that in violent interactions, it is precisely this kind of rapid, almost automatic reaction that occurs before the perpetrator is able to verbalize his or her feelings.

Silent Moments and Pauses Build Space for Talking About the Most Difficult Experiences

We have also investigated the relationship between speech prosody and the processing of emotional experiences in therapy (Itävuori et al., 2015; Kykyri et al., 2017). It was found that a change in speech prosody is a key factor in dealing with difficult emotional experiences. Here, therapists seem to play a key role. In individual psychotherapy situation, the change in speech prosody appeared to be related to both how the client experienced the great sadness associated with the situation they were talking about and the meaning that was constructed for it. When the therapist's speech became quieter, including meaningful pauses, this seemed to contribute to the client's ability to continue talking about the sad experience she was talking about for the first time. When the therapist repeated what he had heard in slightly different words than the client, the stress experienced by the client increased dramatically and decreased when she tearfully said that this was the meaning that this matter had for her. It seemed that the concrete act—putting words to the emotional experience—helped her to reduce the stress she was experiencing and to understand more about this difficult and sad experience she had talked about before. I describe this discussion in Chap. 10.

Change After, Not at the Time of Affective Arousal

Overall, the key conclusion was that in order to understand the synchronicity between clients and therapists, it is important to analyze several data channels simultaneously (Seikkula et al., 2018). In particular, sympathetic nervous system stimulation in the same direction seems to occur at the moment of some specific topics of conversation and modes of dialogue. It is therefore important to understand what people are talking about and how they are speaking at any given moment and to study both the sympathetic nervous system's stimulation at these moments by observing the electrical conductivity of the skin and the parasympathetic nervous system's activity based on heart rate variations. In addition, the participants in the conversation will tune in to each other through body movements and facial expressions. The nervous system is thus part of the overall interaction, reacting to what it is experiencing and also triggering initiatives to which the others present respond. For example, if a speaker is moved while speaking, his voice becomes muffled and he starts to tear up, the listeners immediately react, first with a reaction from their own autonomic nervous system and then, gradually, with conscious thoughts. The autonomic nervous system, like the rest of the human nervous system, is not the cause of behavior, but part of the flow of experience.

An important observation for psychotherapy was the notion that the therapeutic dialogical change occurred after the autonomic nervous system was aroused, not at the moment of arousal. First, the sympathetic nervous system was activated when talking about an important emotive topic and the dialogical encounter with the other started afterwards (Haapanen & Niemi, 2016). For a therapeutic conversation, this means that it is important to first give space to the emerging emotional experience—to be present with the emotional state—and only after the arousal begins to discuss the meaning, explanations, and interpretations of that emerging experience.

Father's Death in the Memory of the Body

I will present a short discussion episode from the second session of couple's therapy. This example illustrates the synchronicity of a very strong emotional response and the autonomic nervous system. Lasse and Heli came to couples therapy because of Lasse's violent behavior. The violence had started after the death of Lasse's father 2 years earlier. Lasse's father had been practically a single parent since the parents' divorce. At this point in the conversation, therapist 2 asks what the father would have said if he had heard the conversation. In dialogical work, this kind of question is very common because it invites the inner voices of the participant into the dialogue.

Lasse: ((sobs)).

T2: I wonder what the father would have said.hh ((pointing to the air)) if (.) he (.) had heard this!

Lasse: ((dry tears))

T2: The conversation (.) we're having, I wonder what he would say ((voice softens)) (2) if he had been here with us (1) and listened to us (1)!

Lasse: I don't know ((shaking his head, crying))

T2: Mm.

(3)

T2: Would he have had any advice to give (.) ((shows his hand))?

Lasse: ((dry tears))

T2: To give you (.)

(3)

Lasse: Maybe just that (.) everything will be fine (1).

T2: ((nods)).hh.

Lasse: Because it's always been done before (.)

T2: That it will all work out, as it has worked out before....

Lasse:Yes..

T2: How would you answer him (.) if he were here to say this (6)

Lasse: I guess all I would do is hug ((scratches his cheek))

T2: Mh (.) mh ((nods)) (2) so (3) mh

Figure 6.1 shows the sympathetic nervous system arousal of all the participants in the discussion, based on skin conductance. At the top, Heli's sympathetic nervous system is quite calm until the question of what Lasse would say to his father, at which point Heli's sympathetic nervous system reacts strongly. His sympathetic response remained high when therapist 1 asked him, after the discussion described above, what he thought of Lasse's response. Although Heli had looked at Lasse very sympathetically, in her response, she was nevertheless critical of Lasse for needing to understand more that this current family was Lasse's most important family.

Lassen's sympathetic nervous system is active all the time and has strong reactions. The highest of these can be seen in the bounded area in Fig. 6.1 when discussing how he would respond to what his father said if he had heard the conversation. The therapist's (T4) sympathetic nervous system reactions follow much of Lassen's nervous system reactions. He was an active participant in the conversation in this topical episode. In contrast, the sympathetic nervous system of the other therapist (T3) is calmed and directed downwards, almost as a mirror image of the reaction of the T4 sympathetic nervous system.

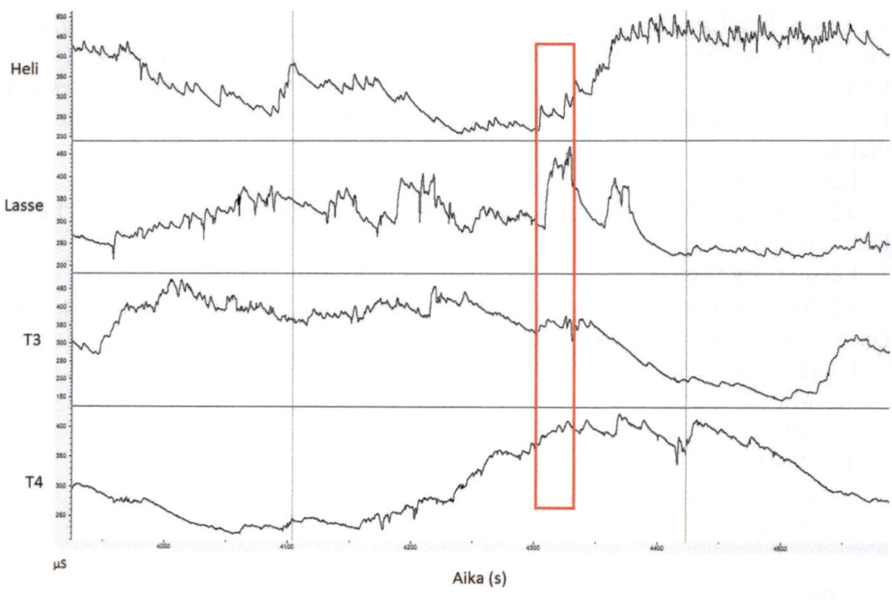

Fig. 6.1 Heli and Lassen's sympathetic nervous system stimulation in couples therapy as measured by skin conductance. Discussion about the death of the father. Isolated part of the passage where the therapist asks how you would respond to the father

This topical episode of conversation is a good illustration of synchronization. Talking about grief provoked a strong reaction, involving both the spouse and one of the therapists. For the other therapist, no stimulation of the sympathetic nervous system occurred at this point. He was more of an observer of the situation. However, this strong sharing of synchrony and emotional experience did not lead to a therapeutic breakthrough, and Heli was still critical of Lasse. Synchronicity per se, therefore, does not yet lead to change.

The therapists' sympathetic nervous system reactions seem almost opposite. Kykyri et al. (2019) studied this particular moment of conversation in detail to determine the therapeutic working relationship. The participants in the therapeutic conversation were interviewed during the day of the conversation. When the therapists, independently of each other, revisited this conversation, they reported that their observations were different. T3 wanted to work on the relationship between clients, while T4 reported that her main focus was on the strong emotional experience. In general, in the session, the therapists' sympathetic nervous system reactions were related to each other. Similarly, the therapists synchronized with each other a lot in their body movements throughout the session. But it was at this particular point that they were both surprised by Lasse's strong emotional response, which T4 wanted to explore and deepen, while T3 hesitated about whether it would be useful. Their different action strategies also seem to be reflected in their different sympathetic nervous system reactions.

Common Regulation of Affective Arousal Arises

Let's look at another example of a therapy conversation where synchronization occurs as the spouses begin to share a common emotional experience (Laitila et al., 2018). The whole conversation is divided into 19 topical episodes for the sake of clarifying the dialogue. In Chap. 9, I describe in more detail the meaning of the topical episode and the DIHC (Dialogical Investigations of Happenings of Change) research methodology used. Figure 6.2 shows how each topic area stimulated the sympathetic nervous system of each participant in the conversation. Where simultaneous firing is observed, the bars for each topic area appear simultaneously. It should be noted that this only describes the synchronization of the autonomic nervous system in the different topical episodes of the conversation. Synchronization occurs in several other areas not considered here (Fig. 6.2). Below, we present excerpts from the discussion in topical Episode 12 and then in topical Episodes 16 and 17. The graph shows that in topical Episode 12, all participants are well attuned. This may be related to the fact that in this topical episode, the therapists talk to each other, which is, therefore, often reflected in an increase in affective arousal and in the stress response experienced by the clients. In topical Episode 16, one of the therapists reacts and in topical Episode 17, he is joined by his wife. These are important points in the construction of the new experience, because the relaxed situation in topical Episode 12 is followed by an intense conversation with affective

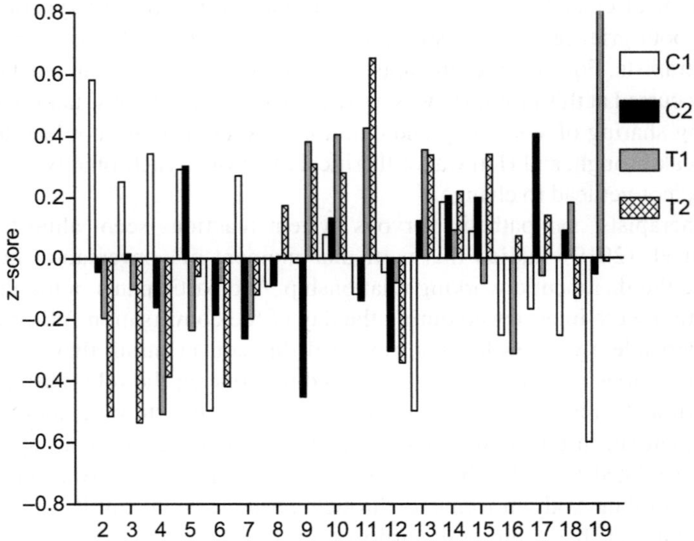

Fig. 6.2 Sympathetic nervous system stimulation of therapists (T1 and T2) and clients (C1 wife and C2 husband) in each of the topical episodes

arousal. This illustrates what was said above that the change comes after the powerful affective arousal.

"So, I'm Not a Traditional Housewife"

The discussion in topical Episode 12 starts by considering the situation of a young family after the birth of a baby. Having lived apart, the couple were very close and shared their affairs with each other. However, the birth of the baby changed the situation fundamentally. The mother became depressed, and the father took on more responsibility for the baby. This made the mother feel like a third wheel. This is discussed at about 43 min into the session.

T1: I mean, when you feel like a third wheel, is there something about feeling like a bad mother...

A (C1): Yes, exactly (.) Mm hm (1) I wonder if guilt also plays a part in it (.) So I'm not the traditional housewife... (2).

[T2: Yes.

A: ...Like...

T1: You're not very... like... keen to change that (.) You said you know you're a lousy.

V: Mm hm.

T1: Mum, if you stayed at home.

[V: Mm.

T1: You're not keen to change that...

V: no

T1: But I hear that you're both building an identity of who I am and what kind of work I should be doing...

M: Mm hm.

T1: In your career and what kind of balance you should make between these different things and what kind of...

M: Yes.

T1: Decisions.

M: ...And we do it personally and it affects our relationship so that you know what to say to each other and how to communicate...

Identity Is a Profound Experience: A Dialogue Between Therapists

T2: ... But Matti (the other therapist), this is also a bit more than identity building, when I remember what we talked about last time, how hard those first months after the baby was born were...

[T1: Yes.

T2: ... So that Eva felt it deeply—of course it's about identity but—but I got the feeling that it was a much deeper experience. Which involves basic questions of existence...

T1: Yes, but I think it involves the basic issues of life...

T1: On how to.

[T2: Okay.

T1: You think about yourself and (.) what you think about yourself and what you become or how I am with others...

[T2: Yeah, yeah, not just how you are socially in situations...

[T1: No, no, more like what I am as a person.

T2: Yes.

T1: Am I a good person or a bad person?

T2: Yes.

T1: ... Am I a good father or am I a good mother?...

[T2: That's right.

T1: ... And how do I get out of this?...

[T2: Yes.

T1: ... And I think they are negotiating these things.

T2: But if I were in this situation as a mother and I found that I couldn't take care of everything because the baby doesn't sleep and I feel very exhausted (.) and then there's the other thing, that the father is taking care (.) That could mean that I might feel even worse (.) because even though I have a good husband, I can't take care of everything. I think there are deep questions all the time.

T1: Yes, and of course these are all very touching feelings...

T2: Yes, yes they are (3).

A: Yes (8).

M: ...Yes...

T2: Yeah..

"What an Impressive Conversation": Spouses' Comments on the Therapists' Dialogue

M: What an, what an impressive conversation, because (2) we came here to talk about us...

T2: Mm hm.

M: .. And still most of our discussion has not been about us (.) but about us as individuals and the baby....

T2: Yes.

M: And (.) it's interesting...

A: It's interesting (.) but it has affected our relationship...

M: Yes (2).

After a strong sympathetic nervous system arousal, the conversation opens up the possibility of talking about something that seems very relevant. Therapist 1 (T1) continues with the wife's earlier experience of being a third wheel and how this affects her identity. When T1 asks, "So you feel like a bad mother," she confirms that she heard Eva's strong comment. When T1 continues by suggesting that this is about a new identity construction, the other therapist (T2) comments to the therapist about her idea of whether this is an even deeper experience than just identity construction related to daily activities. A reflection develops between the therapists on the problems and construction of a new identity on this existential basis. They seem to be on similar wavelengths with slightly different words. Their sympathetic nervous systems were significantly more stimulated than in the average session, but the spouses also listened to their conversation with a relaxed attitude. After the dialogue between the therapists, both spouses say they were impressed by the therapists' conversation because it put their experience into words so well. The husband's active commentary seems to be particularly important, as it shows that he is more involved in the discussion about their relationship in the new situation. This became possible after the therapeutic mutual dialogue.

"I Think We Had Completely Opposite Experiences of This"

The discussion in topical Episode 16 starts about 10 min after the previous episode. For the first time, the husband initiates a new topic of conversation.

M: ((laughing)) Well... I mean, you know the weather, you brought this up (.) and I think it's good that you brought it up (.) I think we had very different experiences in the first year...

T2: Mm mm mm mm.

[M: ... And also the story that I—as you know—for me it was a wonderful experience and I really enjoyed it, although there were parts of it that I didn't like and seeing what he had to go through...

T2: Yes.

M: That there was really bad stuff, not only for her, but for the baby as well, colic and... (1).

T1: Mm.

T2: Yes.

[M: ... But at the same time it was (.) one of the best moments in life (.) if not the best.

[T1: Mm.

M: A moment in my life…

[T1: Mm.

[T2: Yes.

M: And for me it was... it was contradictory (..) to see all that he experienced here....

T2: Yes.

(2)

M2: ....At the time knowing (laughs) that I really liked this...

T1: Yes.

M: Yes (2).

T2: Mm.

A: Yeah, I remember the moment when you said (M smiles) and I was like, what do you think about all this... and he's just going on about how this was the best time of my life...

[T2: Yes.

A: ... And he said and I thought wow he really feels that this was the best time of his life...

[T2: Mm mm.

"The Thing That Broke Our Relationship"

A: ... And I tried to cope with (.) everything. So maybe this is the thing that broke us up, maybe…

[T1: Mm hmm.
[T2: Mm hmm.
A: ....In the first year...
T2: Mm.
[T1: When you said that when you heard what... what does it make you feel?
A: ...That we have two completely opposite experiences of this.
[T1: Yes.
T2: Mm hm.
[A: Yes.
T1: Yes.
[T2: Mm.
T1: .. And that gives you the feeling that your connection has been broken.
A: Yes.
M: Yes... yes.
T1: You are like two completely different experiences at the same time in the same family...
A: Yes.
T1: Experiences together…
A: Yes.
T2: Mm.
(2)
A: And I feel that when we talk about this now, that's really the core of the disconnect (wipes tears with a tissue).
T2: Mm hm.

In this episode, the couple begins to share their most pivotal experience of how they always used to be together, the unit. After the birth of their baby, they have split into individuals, which is the most painful experience. The therapists listen to the development of this experience with compassion and support. There is no need for them to actively comment or ask questions, because sharing this powerful emotional experience is the most important thing right now. The therapists did a great job of giving space to share the emotional state and pain of the birth.

"Earlier We Were Like a Unit"

M: And I think, because before that we all had such similar experiences...
[T1: Mm hm so.
M: Yes.
A: It was like... we were kind of a unit (..) we moved everywhere together...
[T2: Yes.
A: Than experiencing all this newness together.
T2: Yes.
A: ... Life here, its ups and downs and travelling a lot. We were really one powerful unit...

T1: Mm.
T2: Mm.

"The Best Time of My Life"

A: And then came that first year (.) we were (3) like (2), but you must never have said bad things to me (1). I think you only said once that it was the best time of your life...

M: (1) Now I see what it meant to you...
A: ((Swallows)).
T2: Excuse me?
M: I knew how he felt about it...
T2: Uh-huh (.) by saying that, that...
T1: Oh, yes.
[M: I could see it in his face...
[T2: You saw it before you said it?
M: (.) Not really, but anyway it was in that moment (.) when he asked me, and I just said (.)
T2: Yes.
M: ...I said.... and then (1) I could see it right away from his face that it wasn't...
T1: Mm.
T2: Yes.
M: ...Even close (1)...
T1: Yes.
M: Yes (2).
T2: Yes.
(4)
T1: Yes.
M: Yes, that's right.
(3)
A: ((tears))... And that's (.) when you know you're having a gigantic experience (voice breaks).
[T2: Mm.
A: (1) Happening (.) and when we, you know we're hard as a rock together and when this happens (.) then you're like (.) you're two beings apart...
(3)
T2: Yes.
A: A few months after Eva was born, we really, you know, we worked together and (.) even though there were those circumstances, her colic and that state of mind....
[T2: Mm hm.
A: However, we worked very well together...
M: Yes, but then I went back to work...

A: Yes, it was difficult.
(2)
T2: Mm mm.

"Whenever He Was at Work I Was Just at Home"

A: When you were at home it was much easier and when you went to work it became really difficult (turns up his nose).

M: Mm.
(3)
V: Mm mm.
(2)
T2: Mm.
A: Mm... ((wipes his tears)).
(12)
M: ((swallows)).
A: So, oh my god, we're like...(1) we got a nanny (1) ((M swallows)).
T2: Yes.
A: And every time (.) when he was working, and I was just at home....
M: It was really violent....
(...)

A: So mm mm mm (2) and I think a lot about the guilt that I only have.... and we were talking about this last time here, when there's this story about how wonderful it is when you have a baby and you just fall in love with it and la*la*laa*.

During this conversation, the wife and Therapist 1 do not show any stimulation of the sympathetic nervous system, while T2 and the husband react slightly more than the average of the session. Synchronizing pairs are thus formed on the therapist-client axis, and thus, each client receives a response from one therapist in terms of sympathetic nervous system stimulation. This discussion deepens the process begun in the previous passage, in which the man becomes a more active and responsible participant in the marital relationship. It seems that the wife also reacts to this with strong emotional expressions by crying, but at the beginning of the episode, more by listening and occasionally commenting. Gradually, she also began to talk about her experiences in tears.

The snippets above illustrate the way in which sharing is created between spouses and how their bodily reactions are involved in building the possibility of new learning. The intensity of the conversation is also well illustrated by the fact that, at the beginning of the next therapy session, both described how impressed they were with this conversation. They also reported that they liked very much being able to watch snippets of the conversation after the session in the researcher's interview.

In the subjects described here, a lot of body movement synchrony was observed, but this was not directly related to autonomic nervous system stimulation (Nyman-Salonen et al., 2020). For example, one of the therapists (T2) followed the conversation a lot with head nods, and the other a lot by directing his gaze to the speaker. The husband directed a lot of his gaze to his wife, who, in turn, looked more at the therapists. Body movements increased precisely in the key areas of the conversation described here. It seems that the different aspects of bodily synchrony function independently in relation to each other but are nevertheless related to the emotional experience of what it is spoken about.

The Body As a Part of Psychotherapy and Other Encounters

We can reflect on the surprising initial findings of our research and to look what the findings of other studies have to offer to psychological support, including psychotherapy. In the case of embodiment, I have described here only a very small part of the whole. What has not been discussed above is how the human central nervous system—that is, brain activity—is involved in processing emotional sensations, giving meaning to them and synchronizing the present. This is an even greater challenge for research than studying the autonomic nervous system in a live interaction situation. For brain research, laboratory-like research situations can be constructed in which study participants are exposed to specific stimuli, and then the response of a precisely activated brain area is studied. But as noted above, it may be that such a research design may not accurately capture the basic pulse of life. In practice, in everyday life, meanings are created in an ever-flowing interaction, both on the basis of the visceral messages of one's own body and through the influence of and influence on people present in a social situation. Thus, for example, it is not yet methodologically feasible to perform brain imaging in such an interactive situation, so such knowledge is very preliminary.

Porges (2011) has done significant work on the connection between emotions and the brain by creating the so-called polyvagal theory. Humans are most vulnerable to external influences through the autonomic nervous system. The heart is probably our most important internal organ in regulating autonomic nervous system function. For example, emotional sensations are generated by changes in heart rate and blood pressure. Porges has studied, in particular, how the vagal nerve connects the heart and the brain and how these are connected to the rest of the body. By understanding how the vagus nerve works, we can understand how emotional states in the brain always have meanings in relation to the rest of the body and the social situation. In one example, Porges explains that in an interactive situation; by looking down, the speaker or listener regulates their own shame or anger. This is often not put into words, but this gesture of interaction is, of course, very powerful and easily noticeable. Thus, this gesture is received and influences the response of the other participant, which in turn influences the speaker's experience of the situation and the progress of the dialogue between them. All this can happen in a very short time, so that no participant has time to give it any conscious narrative meaning, but it affects everyone's experience.

According to Trevarthen, a characteristic of human life is the telling of stories. Even a small baby starts telling stories. At first, of course, these stories are not stories in words, but the baby uses a wide variety of vocalizations, movements, gestures, looks, smiles, and cries to tell his stories to his parents and others. The baby tells stories with his body, and naturally, the response he receives either encourages him to go further or causes him to become defensive. This is a very similar activity to the stories told by an adult human being, even though they take place in spoken language.

What we have described so far can already be summarized in a few guidelines on what to consider in a psychotherapy situation, at least, in order to make the best use of the full involvement of clients and therapists.

1. It is important to accept the psychic as the embodied mind, so that we meet people as a whole without dividing them into body and soul. There are already many examples of this in various psychotherapeutic methods. For example, mindfulness exercises are already widely used in psychotherapists' training and clinical work.
2. It is important to understand human life as a whole, as part of an active network of relationships, its relationality, and its construction of relationships. The embodiment emphasizes, in particular, the importance of shared common emotional experiences. This brings more felt emotions into the therapy session. Often, just experiencing emotional experiences together can be a healing experience, while at other times, it is worthwhile to try to construct their verbal meaning. This can be challenging for therapists, as many therapy methods in the past have emphasized the importance of neutrality and not of bringing up one's own emotional experiences of therapists, such as being moved.
3. It is important to tolerate uncertainty and tolerate silence by allowing more time for clients to bring up previously unspoken issues and their related unforeseen emotional experiences.
4. It is important to understand embodiment as a whole human being, so that the functions of the mind are not reduced to those of the brain. The brain is an integral part of emotional experience and meaning-making, but it can be risky to explain a particular emotional state or mental health problem by a disorder in one brain area. For example, the cause of a psychotic experience cannot be attributed to a specific brain dysfunction, but it is important to understand brain function as part of a holistic bodily response to relational situations.

Taking these issues into account in psychotherapy and psychological encounters will change the way we work. I have often found that this allows for more psychotherapy, especially for men. A common developmental psychological and clinical observation is that women develop better at expressing their own emotional experiences in words and in conversation. An assumption has been that men generally seem to have fewer words, and, therefore, may benefit less from psychotherapy. But if we accept emotional experiences as one way of expressing themselves, men can become more involved, even if they have no words to describe their own experiences. The same goes for any who is not so used to formulating her or his emotional experiences into spoken narratives. Often in family therapy, or even in wider social network meetings, those who do not are so used to speaking can experience very strong emotions. When these feelings are acknowledged and responded to, it can already be a healing experience, encouraging them to move forward in talking about difficult issues. This was well illustrated in the two therapy sessions above. Initially, only the wife brought up the topics of discussion. After a discussion between the therapists, the husband became active and spoke for the first time about his own feelings and emotions.

References

Haapanen, K., & Niemi, P. (2016). *Moments of change in multidisciplinary therapy dialogues in couples therapy University of Jyväskylä, Department of Psychology, Jyväskylä*. Jyväskylä Psychology Department, Jyväskylä University of Psychology.

Itävuori, S., Korvela, E., Karvonen, A., Penttonen, M., Kaartinen, J., Kykyri, V. L., & Seikkula, J. (2015). The significance of silent moments in creating words for the not-yet-spoken experiences in threat of divorce. *Psychology, 6*, 1360–1372. Published Online August 2015 in SciRes.

Karvonen, A., Kykyri, V. L., Kaartinen, J., Penttonen, M., & Seikkula, J. (2016). Sympathetic nervous system synchrony in couple therapy. *Journal of Marital and Family Therapy, 42*(3), 383–395.

Kykyri, V. L., Karvonen, A., Wahlström, J., Kaartinen, J., Penttonen, M., & Seikkula, J. (2017). Soft prosody and embodied attunement in therapeutic interaction: A multimethod case study of a moment of change. *Journal of Constructivist Psychology, 30*(3), 211–234. https://doi.org/10.1080/10720537.2016.1183538

Kykyri, V.-L., Tourunen, A., Nyman-Salonen, P., Kurri, K., Wahlström, J., Kaartinen, J., Penttonen, M., & Seikkula, J. (2019). Alliance formations in couple therapy - a multi-modal and multimethod study. *Journal of Couple and Relationship Therapy., 18*, 189–222. https://doi.org/10.1080/15332691.2018.1551166

Laitila, A., Vall, B., Penttonen, M., Kykyri, V.-L., Karvonen, A., Tsatsishvili, V., Kaartinen, J., & Seikkula, J. (2018). The added value of studying embodied responses in couple therapy research: A case study. *Family Process, 58*, 669–684.

Nyman-Salonen, P., Vall, B., Laitila, A., Borcsa, M., Penttonen, M., Tourunen, A., Kykyri, V.-L., Kaartinen, J., Tsatsishvili, V., & Seikkula, J. (2020). Significant moments in a couple therapy session: Towards the integration of different modalities of analysis. In M. Ochs, M. Borcsa, & J. Schweitzer (Eds.), *Systemic research in individual, couple and family therapy and counseling* (pp. 55–74). Springer.

Päivinen, H., Holma, J., Karvonen, A., Kykyri, V. L., Tsatsishvili, V., Kaartinen, J., Penttonen, M., & Seikkula, J. (2016). Affective arousal during blaming in couple therapy: Combining analyses of verbal discourse and physiological responses in two case studies. *Contemporary Family Therapy, 38*, 373–384. https://doi.org/10.1007/s10591-016-9393-7

Porges, S. (2011). *The polyvagal theory: Neurophysiological foundations of emotions, attachment, communication, self-regulation*. Norton.

Seikkula, J., Karvonen, A., Kykyri, V. L., Kaartinen, J., & Penttonen, M. (2015). The embodied attunement of therapists and a couple within dialogical psychotherapy: An introduction to the relational mind research project. *Family Process, 54*, 703–715.

Seikkula, J., Karvonen, A., Kykyri, V. L., Penttonen, M., & Nyman-Salonen, P. (2018). The relational mind in couple therapy: A Bateson-inspired view of human life as an embodied stream. *Family Process, 57*(4), 855–866.

Chapter 7
Psychotic Behavior Is a Part of Dialogue, Not a Pathology

Introduction

In the previous chapters, we have explored the transformation brought about by a dialogical conception of the human being. My basic assumption is that the extraordinary results of dialogical practice in the treatment of the most severe mental health problems are related to its ability to access essential resources of the person affected and his or her family—resources that cannot be seen in a pathological framework focused solely on symptoms. It is therefore worth asking what this new view of the human being means in the most difficult psychological crises, such as psychotic problems. Dialogical practice makes it possible to understand psychotic behavior as one possible response to extreme stress. Psychosis is not a psychopathological condition or illness, but an active function of the human mind in an extreme situation. The person having psychotic experiences is not a powerless victim of his or her illness; they have their own resources for coping with the crisis. Relying on these resources—both in the individual and their loved ones—has also contributed significantly to reducing the use of neuroleptic medication and preventing its side effects. Dialogue helps to mobilize clients' resources in a psychotic crisis.

Psychosis as a Psychopathology: Peoples' Own Resources Disappear

Mental disorders are commonly seen as psychopathologies. According to this perspective, diagnostic category reflects a specific construction of the mind. From a medical point of view, classifying mental health problems into diagnoses makes sense. I also believe it is important to recognize different types of problems during conversations with those seeking help and their families. For instance, it is important to recognize if someone has stopped eating (an "eating disorder"), or is so

J. Seikkula, *Why Dialogue Does Cure*,
https://doi.org/10.1007/978-3-031-91294-8_7

depressed that they are possibly thinking about suicide. Similarly, it is important to recognize if someone in the present conversation starts talking about phenomena that I think include delusions or hallucinations as psychotic experiences. In this case, I know that not everything will be said explicitely in this discussion, but that there will also be voices involved whose message is very difficult to formulate in unambiguous terms. When talking about eating problems or depression, it is important to recognize that these issues, if left untreated, can become life-threatening. There is nothing wrong in identifying problems; doing so is an important part of helping people in the most difficult crises.

Diagnoses become a problem when they are seen as determinants for organizing the therapy of mental health problems. If someone's mental state is seen as a pathological problem, it becomes difficult to find the resources needed to solve the problems, because their mind is in a pathological state.

The dialogical approach has changed my own understanding of mental health problems in a very fundamental way. In this chapter, my aim is to challenge strong pathological thinking and describe the possibilities of seeing the most difficult mental health problems as an active functioning of the mind under insurmountable stress. It is particularly important to reconsider how we understand psychosis and schizophrenia, as our conception of these phenomena reveals much about our broader understanding of the human condition. Currently, there is far too little reflection on our understanding of the human being, which has given rise to the uncritical adoption of very strange and damaging treatment recommendations that are supposedly based on scientific evidence. The over-pathologization of mental health problems fixes the identity of a person as a patient and reduces the ability of their family and networks to influence the course of the so-called "illness."

Pathological thinking is also deeply rooted in other sciences. In philosophy, for example, mental health problems are often described as pathological categories. Phenomenology, as a philosophical orientation, has been very interested in anomalies of states of mind. In general, phenomenology is interested in the perspective of the person experiencing psychosis—the individual as experiencer. But for me, the human mind is not something possessed by the individual, but is realized in a flow of relationships—best realized in responsive actions in multi-actor situations in real interactions in real-life situations. Philosophical accounts often treat schizophrenia or psychosis as a permanent characteristic of a person, involving specific forms of perception, reasoning, and sensing. For example, Abettan (2015), in his otherwise important study of phenomenology in psychiatry, notes how most attempts have failed because they did not incorporate the core of phenomenology: the inclusion of the individual's own unique experience in describing psychiatric phenomena. At the end of his study, he asks, "Is phenomenology really approaching pathological states of mind?" (p. 538), suggesting that doing is needed to understand schizophrenia. So, according to him too, it is a pathological state of mind.

Mental Symptoms Indicate an Active Mind

But what if psychotic behavior is not a "pathological state of mind." A more constructive perspective for helping is to consider all human mental activity as a response to life events. Psychological symptoms are also responses to life, not signs of illness. Often even the opposite: they show the mind's active capacity to protect itself in times of stress. Psychic work is the body's response to everything that happens in a continuous flow, which cannot be stopped or isolated from its connections for observation. The phenomenologist Maurice Merleau-Ponty (Carman, 2008) described human existence as bodily movements that create our perspective on the world. Levinas (1985) was interested in the human mind in relationships, where the Other always awaits our response—it cannot be escaped. It is in this response that the psychic mind of our action is born. Psychotic behavior is no different from this in any way; it is one way of responding to the Other. Often, the psychotic response involves an attempt to withdraw or isolate oneself from relationships that are perceived as too close or pervasive.

What I write here is based on my own clinical experiences over 40 years of helping people who have had psychotic experiences and their families, and my research on Open Dialogue and psychotic problems. Several studies have found that Open Dialogue has produced unprecedented results in the treatment of psychotic patients (see Chap. 1). For example, a 19-year follow-up found that psychotic patients treated in Open Dialogue were twice as likely to be employed as those receiving conventional treatment. Patients in Open Dialogue used significantly fewer treatment services and less psychotropic medication compared to patients treated in the rest of the country. This long-term follow-up showed that the dialogical approach used some 20 years ago had far-reaching effects—not only on individual's life, enabling them to remain employed and independent of treatment—but also on societal costs, such as reduced hospitalization and medication. It is important to consider how a new understanding of psychotic problems is linked to better treatment outcomes.

Psychosis is not a separate category; a person who has psychotic experiences is not qualitatively different from someone who does not. Moncrieff and Leo (2010) noted that no study has shown that all psychotic patients exhibit specific changes in their brains compared to non-psychotic individuals. Psychotic behavior is not related to a specific structural feature but emerges from a wide range of experiences and developmental trajectories. All people engage in relational responses in their own unique way. In extremely stressful situations, a psychotic response is possible for anyone—not just for those with a particular personality structure or vulnerability.

Rather than seeing psychotic behavior as an abnormality or structural defect, it can be seen as an active attempt by the embodied mind to cope with extreme stress. Psychotic experiences are emotional experiences of the body–mind. People who have such experiences are often unable to describe their emotional experiences explicitly. For example, by stating that "I began to hear my mother's voice when I realized the conflict we were experiencing in our family." Instead, she may experience overwhelming bodily arousal that creates a huge emotional storm. She begins to hallucinate that she cannot perceive with her senses. In this way, her mind is actively processing unbearable stress through the voice she hears. In her hallucination or paranoid delusion, she expresses something that has actually happened—though metaphorically—through language that cannot be tied directly to a single clear event or experience. Hallucination is a powerful emotion through which a person actively defends themselves against an even more terrible experience. Some researchers (Holma & Aaltonen, 1997) have argued that this reflects the pre-narrative nature of psychotic behavior—we are working through experiences for which there is not (yet) a narrative in words, but which manifest as intense sensations or feelings in our bodies. This is not a psychiatric illness, but a possible and necessary way for all of us to protect ourselves when under extreme pressure. It is the mind's active way of defending itself against this insurmountable pressure.

Psychological Stress Cuts Off the Internal Dialogue

One dimension of psychotic experience is the disruption of internal dialogue between different voices, resulting in disconnected and fragmented experiences. This lack of integration may lead to extreme emotional agitation, making our experiences feel alien—outside of ourselves. Indeed, what we experience may seem to be part of an external observer, somehow connected to the present moment. Psychotic perception involves two important aspects. First is the breakdown in distinguishing between self and other in our perception of reality—though this covers only a small part of our perceptions. The second aspect involves how, through observing external reality, I perceive myself as part of it. For example, how do I explain a sound I hear in the room when I cannot see its source? If I explain it as a hallucination, I can control my experience, at least to some extent. If, on the other hand, I explain it as being due to, say, supernatural abilities or a message sent to me by other people, the experience becomes psychotic, and the power of action is transferred to this external agent. *If this happens, it is very important that the people present—such as therapists—accept me with this experience, without defining me as ill.* Their acceptance and associated recognition of my difficult situation can enhance my ability to regain control over my mind. It can also strengthen my social connections, thereby reinforcing my sense of reality and my chances of returning to a world of experience without psychotic experiences. The basic premise of all this is that such experiences are not signs of illness, but the mind's active response to extreme pressure. In discussion, this means that phenomena are discussed as normal responses to this kind of conflict or pressure, not as symptoms of sickness or strangeness.

Karon and Vandenbos (1981) and Karon (2003) have stated that in psychotic behavior, a person deals with experiences of horror that, because of the massive emotional turmoil they contain, could not be put into an unambiguous narrative.

These experiences have no language other than hallucinations and delusions, and in a dialogical approach, putting such hallucinations or delusions into words can be the beginning of putting one's own experiences into understandable and processable narratives. According to Karon, psychotic experiences are associated with the terror of death, and delusions serve as defenses against this terror. However, they are not just hallucinations or delusions—the person is speaking about something important that has really happened.

Psychotic Experience Can Help to Deal with Difficult Memories

However, terrible or traumatic experiences in an individual's past life do not trigger psychotic behavior and are therefore not the cause of psychotic behavior. In a psychotic experience, people may recount events that happened decades earlier. The implicit memories of those events are evoked in the current interaction and are responses to current emotional experiences. Psychotic reactions can be seen as attempts to make sense of one's own experiences and to cope with such difficult experiences for which it has been impossible to construct a coherent narrative. The stressful situation of the moment may in some ways resemble the original horrific experience and thus actualize memories without the person being aware of the relationship between the two events at different times. The recollection can occur from a very small cue, for example, just the sensation of a similar smell or color, or the reliving of a similar unpleasant emotional experience in the current conversation.

This is illustrated by the case of a mother who, in a psychotic experience, feared that her husband was drug-addicted and was going to kill her. At the therapy meeting, she told the doctor that 16 years ago she had been cohabiting with a drug addict. In his drug addiction, her partner had repeatedly beaten her. She had never revealed this horrific experience to anyone. During their two-year relationship, she had truly lived in fear of death. Two months before her first psychotic episode, he called her for the first time in 12 years. She said that when she heard his voice on the phone, she couldn't say anything; she just shook. Her body remembered all the horror of the death her partner had caused with his violence. The fear she felt with her current husband was psychotic; he had no intention of coming to kill her. But at the same time, she was telling about something that really had happened in her life. Her psychotic experience was a reference to her relationship with a man who had repeatedly threatened her life with violence. Thus, the experience in her body's memory was real, but it appeared to be spoken as if in a metaphorical way. It was in this conversation that she for the first time spoke of this terrible violence she had experienced several years earlier. It is remarkable that only her psychotic experience made it possible for her to talk about such an important experience in her life.

Such serious experiences of victimhood are not stored in the part of memory where we can recall our experiences with unambiguous narratives. Van der Kolk et al. (2006) have described how traumatic horror experiences can begin to live in the mind as flashbacks without the person being able to identify their source. They can also take the form of dissociative experiences that often closely resemble psychotic phenomena (Read et al., 2004). Studies have found that 60% of men and 69% of women experienced sexual or physical abuse in childhood. These experiences are therefore very real, not just meaningless mental productions.

Karon and Vandenbos saw hallucinations as narratives of real-life events involving the horror of death as experienced. It is very important that the therapist understands that the ones having psychotic experiences are talking about their real experiences and not just about meaningless hallucinations. In their book, for example, they describe a young man who suddenly began to speak Latin, although he was not known to have studied Latin. Instead of treating this as an insignificant coincidence, the therapist began to ask whether the young man had any experience of church. In the course of the therapy, it emerged that he had indeed been a choirboy in a Catholic church as a teenager, and later it emerged that he had been sexually abused by a parish priest.

As a starting point for successful therapy, Karon and Vandenbos suggest that the psychotherapist should take a strong position by supporting the patient against the horror of death by promising not to let anyone harm the patient. From a dialogical point of view, their descriptions of the link between psychotic experiences and real-life events are very useful. We can see delusional experiences as inner voices and develop a dialogue between these different voices. Unfortunately, their descriptions of horizontal (i.e. interpersonal) polyphony are not very useful, because they tend to see the mother—and the family in general—as the cause of psychotic problems. Because of this assumption, they did not get on well with the family and suggested family meetings with another therapist. As I have often said, one of the basic assumptions of a dialogical approach is that we give up diagnosing and fault-finding for clients and their families and instead accept them just as they are. This seems to provide the best starting point for a new dialogue in which both the psychotic experiencer at the center of concern and his or her family members begin to be heard and accepted. In this way, new forms of communication can begin to be learned that were previously not possible within the family.

Psychotic Behavior as an Embodied Activity

A psychotic experience involves a lot of physical experiences. Several bodily reactions have been observed in hallucinations and other psychotic experiences (Lysaker & Lysaker, 2004; Mitropoulos, 2020). In both psychotic hallucinations and dissociative reactions, individuals may experience strange bodily sensations for no apparent reason, for example, a smell or unexplained pain in some parts of the body. A stressful current life situation activates previous similar affective memories in the body. When dealing with an overwhelming emotional turmoil, the embodied mind creates hallucinations or delusions instead of clear and unambiguous memories.

The body speaks through metaphors, creating narratives of our experiences. When another person first hears the content of the hallucinations, they may seem impossible to understand because the person is experiencing the actual sounds and events as if from outside themselves. If the clinicians present do not accept the person's reality, they have fewer opportunities to explore their own experiences, which undermines their ability to control their own behavior (Roe & Davidson, 2005).

Sometimes psychotic experiences and forms of communication become so powerful that they take over the person's perceptual world. Other voices that are constructive and necessary to adapt to the social situation are silenced, and the dialogue between the different voices stops. The focus on symptoms in treatment may exacerbate this situation, as the over-pathologization of the problem and the associated treatment practices reduce the ability of the diagnosed person to take greater control of their own life. Stating that psychosis is a brain disorder that has nothing to do with a person's real-life experiences, we reduce their ability to integrate those experiences. These types of remarks further limit the dialogue with others and thus limit the opportunities for self-understanding and action (Avdi et al., 2015).

For someone experiencing a psychotic crisis, it can help to look at delusions and hallucinations as feelings. Emotions are the body's responses, and emotions help the body restore homeostasis if we experience a threat from inside or outside the body. Emotions—such as anxiety, panic reactions, or depressed moods—are a natural part of life in different circumstances. They trigger our natural defense system and are vital to the body's defense mechanisms. In extreme situations, they can become problematic, and emotions begin to block constructive responses to everyday stress. When this happens, a person can be diagnosed as suffering from anxiety, panic disorder or depression. A similar phenomenon occurs in the area of delusions and hallucinations. Hallucinations are the embodied mind's responses and attempts to adapt to extreme stress, especially in situations where there are multiple stressors acting simultaneously (Karon & Vandenbos, 1981).

We can all experience hallucinations, often in the extreme situations of normal life. For example, a person may hear the voice of a loved one who has died suddenly and have no difficulty understanding the experience as being related to grief. The emotions are trying to restore homeostasis and rescue oneself from the pain of loss. But if the stress continues to increase, the person may lose touch with reality testing and interpret their own emotional experiences. This can develop into a psychotic experience. They may experience the voice of a deceased loved one in both their internal and external life, and no longer understand the connection between this experience and their grief. The person has lost the ability to understand the symbolic meaning of this hallucination and begins to believe it to be true, as if the dead person were really speaking in their head.

Hallucinations and delusions are expressions of the human emotional system that adapt to extreme stress and are not symptoms of a neurobiological disease, although emotional reactions naturally contain strong physical elements. The vast majority of delusions, for example, occur in people who never seek psychiatric treatment because they do not need it (de Leede-Smith & Barkus, 2014). The main aim of therapy is to help people better understand their reactions and how they relate to their current and past experiences. Therefore, in therapy, we can think about ways in which emotional upsets may be linked to depression or panic attacks. Similarly, we can consider the meaning of an experience that has developed into psychosis and how it relates to our own life events. Neither psychosis nor schizophrenia are psychopathological conditions; the production of psychotic responses under extreme stress is a sign of a functioning mind that finds ways to defend itself and restore the organism's homeostasis. It is important to recognize that in a psychotic experience, a person may begin to develop non-functional ways of dealing with their problem, which can then develop into a life-limiting situation.

Dialogues on Psychotic Experiences

In Open Dialogues, we are used to engage in dialogue with people experiencing psychotic phenomena. In a therapy meeting—which includes the team, the person at the center of concern, their family, and possibly others—the unique way of seeing of the problem is the primary focus. Each discussion is always unique and is based on how each participant perceives the issue. The therapists—there are more than one—adapt their way of speaking to the individual and unique needs of each patient and their family, taking into account that each discussion creates a new language. What has been discussed before does not accumulate as an agenda for a meeting. New meanings emerge with each conversation, even if the family has attended several times already. Each person present speaks in their own voice, which must be respected. Listening and responding becomes the most important part of dialogical interaction, which is much more important than the interview approach.

In a therapy session with a person experiencing psychosis, it is important to accept their hallucinations or delusions as voices among others. These are not challenged, for example, by stating that they are part of the illness. On the contrary, the person is encouraged to talk more about their experiences. The aim of Open Dialogue is to enable participants to build a new language to express and discuss together the most difficult events in their lives. The events can be of any type and could have happened at any time; the goal is not to find the exact original experiences. Regardless of previous experiences, it is important to take hallucinations seriously and avoid challenging the patient's reality, particularly during a crisis and in the early stages of treatment. Instead, the therapist could ask: "Did I hear you correctly when you said that you control your neighbor's thoughts? Could you tell me more about this?" Other members of the network might then be asked, "What do others think about this? How do you understand what M is saying?" The aim is to bring forth a range of perceptions about the issues under discussion, including the psychotic experience. As Trimble (2000) stated "building trust in the regulation of interpersonal emotional experience allows others to influence us in a dialogical relationship."

Building trust by listening to everyone's voice is a key principle. This is profoundly different from the experiences many people report from hospital treatment.

Once, a young man who had been hospitalized for the third time due to psychosis asked us for a discussion with his family. His parents had been disappointed by a family meeting at the hospital the previous day. He said that his parents were willing to come for a discussion, even though they had been divorced for 20 years and had no connection with each other—in fact, he said they could not tolerate each other in the same room. I thought it was important to build trust with everyone, so I suggested that we do not start directly with a joint session. Instead, we held separate conversations: the first with him, his younger brother, and their mother; the second with the brothers and their father; and only the third with all four together. That third meeting—their first joint session—was extremely emotionally charged. The younger brother admitted that he was terrified of this conversation, saying it should have taken place 20 years ago when their parents separated. A moment later, the mother said the same. During the conversation, the younger brother raised difficult issues from their childhood. He talked about the problems between the parents and their inability to care for their children, and he was particularly critical of his father for their childhood experiences.

During the discussion, the father appeared very rigid—both mentally and in how he sat—but he listened to the children's criticism. When asked for his thoughts, he said he was sorry for what they had experienced and that it was never his intention to harm them. I also asked him if he was comfortable continuing the conversation, and he replied that it was the right thing to do and that now was the time to talk. Toward the end of the therapy meeting, the atmosphere became calmer, and the family even joked about their history. When we asked for their comments on the conversation at the end of the discussion, they all said they were surprised at how different this conversation had been compared to the hospital meeting. They felt that the doctor in charge in the hospital seemed only interested in finding out how disturbing the young man was, and in diagnosing the family as problematic. In contrast, during our joint dialogical therapy meeting, they all felt heard and respected, despite having very different opinions. They repeated this same experience at the end of every conversation during our one-and-a-half-year therapy relationship. Respecting and listening to others are the main aim of dialogical work, whereas in psychiatric treatment, the aim is often to find out "how crazy the other person is" or to uncover what the family's problems are—if the family is interested in meeting at all.

In a therapy session, the psychotic person seems to start talking in a psychotic way when discussing the most sensitive and relevant experiences that do not have any other words to deal with. Perhaps it is at this moment that something fundamental about a still unspoken experience is touched upon. It is important that therapists take advantage of the opportunity that presents itself to begin talking about the most difficult experiences. For example, a therapist might ask, "What did I say that might have led you to speak in that way?" or, "What were we talking about when M started talking about how a voice was controlling her?"

The basic idea in a therapy meeting is that staff allow the patient and their network to lead in determining the content of the discussion. The therapist's main role is to ensure that the expressions of family members are responded to in the dialogue, through which the different participants are given the opportunity for new understanding. One way of responding is to initiate reflective discussions among the members of the working group. This can be done by asking kindly for permission: "Could you wait a moment so we can discuss what has come to our minds? Afterward, we will ask for comments on what we said." In most cases, participants listen closely to how the clinicians have understood their problems.

Some Simple Guidelines for Dialogue

In dialogical practice, the main aim of therapeutic conversations is to create a dialogue both between the participants and the inner voices of the participants themselves. Thus, participants are encouraged to bring forward different perspectives rather than a single common opinion, promoting reflection. This, in turn, contributes to an exploration of different dimensions of issues and different voices. It opens the way for listening to the experiences of other family members in difficult life situations. Family members may be surprised by each other's views—for example, when siblings remember some childhood experiences in very different ways. If they themselves are respected and heard in this discussion, they will become more open to hearing other family members' experiences. This happened, for example, in the conversation I described earlier, where a younger brother's criticism of his father came as a surprise to his brother, who was a patient in hospital. In turn, openness to new voices can increase agency and the ability to influence one's own life by understanding one's own views and position in relation to other family members.

For clinicians, the starting point is unconditional acceptance of the other, which is often difficult between family members in times of crisis. This is particularly acute in a psychotic crisis, when one family member seems to be talking about a completely different reality, as if in a foreign language. In these dialogues, we do not question the other's expression but rather encourage them to speak more about their experience, so that we can better understand their perspective and the way others relate to it. There is no room in a dialogue to begin teaching the person that their (psychotic) speech is part of an illness and not of reality.

Here are some more specific guidelines for dialogue.

Focus Consistently on Relationships

The human-relations perspective applies equally to horizontal and vertical voices (Haarakangas, 1997). By horizontal voices, we mean the conversation between those present in the room. A key challenge for clinicians is how to create an atmosphere in which everyone feels treated equally, so that everyone's opinions are respected. Everyone is encouraged to participate in the discussion, speaking as much as they want and commenting on others' contribution. In an acute crisis, the discussion may start with a psychotic person, who should be listened to with curiosity. At the same time, it is important to observe how others react to this seemingly strange speech. We can ask how they feel in response to what is being said. It often seems important to ask specifically what feelings the speech evokes, rather than encouraging debate about whether an experience is right or wrong. In this way, clinicians can create opportunities for connections between family members and prevent the isolation that often seems almost automatically associated with a psychotic experience.

The second area of polyphony is the internal, vertical voice of each participant. It is very important to be sensitive to the fact that the person with psychosis is not really psychotic all the time or in every topic of conversation, but engages in a very diverse way, like anyone else. Both forms of speech—conventional and psychotic—are equally acceptable and will be responded to. Other family members also experience a wide range of, at times conflicting, feelings. While they may express very negative comments about the person in crisis, they also have a deep concern and affection for them. Everyone should be encouraged to talk about life in general, not just the crisis that has brought them together.

Respecting the Psychotic Experience Unconditionally

In a psychotic crisis, the aim is not to change the psychotic person's experience but to be deeply curious about it. One of the key aims of a dialogical conversation is to make space for the speaker to hear themselves, through respectful responses from the clinicians. At the beginning of a crisis conversation, it is unlikely that a person experiencing psychosis will be able to reflect on their experiences. When someone starts talking psychotically, it is often because we are touching on something deeply painful or traumatic—something for which they have no other words. If, at that moment, we begin to orient them to reality, we increase the risk that they will not be unable to reflect later on how psychotic experience connects to the painful life experiences. If we instead accept what they are saying, we encourage them to talk more about their delusions and hallucinations and begin to construct a more understandable narrative of what is happening in their life.

In the middle of a crisis, most people believe their delusions to be real, and it is very important at that moment to stop any other conversation and encourage them to tell more. I might say, "Wait a minute—did I hear you say you were on a program? Can you tell me more about that? When did it start? Is it the same throughout the day?" These are just examples of how we can begin to discuss what seems like very strange experiences in everyday language, rather than taking them as pathological and signs of illness as our basic assumption. Accepting the person unconditionally, even in psychosis, is a very challenging practice for clinicians, but its aim is to promote a sense of acceptance.

During the therapeutic process, people may begin to think that the voices they hear may not be real, but are sensations of their own. At this point—though still hearing voices—they are no longer psychotic. This also allows for a very different kind of dialogue. For example, in one therapy process, a person told of hearing the voice of an aunt who strongly criticized her religion. Initially, she believed that her aunt had developed some very sophisticated method of entering her room without permission. Over time, she began to consider that the voice was not really controlling her, but the reflection of the conflict between her and her family over religion than actual intrusion.

Whether it is an acute or a long-term psychotic problem, the main guiding principle is to talk with the person, not to the "psychotic patient." If we are oriented to talk with the psychotic patient, our attention is easily drawn to the problematic aspects of behavior, reinforcing a psychopathological thinking. Do not look for pathological features in the person or their family! This is a central guideline for dialogical therapy. The aim is to mobilize the resources of the person who needs help, which are often already present but obstructed by crisis.

Attention to the Emotional Experience of Lived Things

People with psychotic experiences may talk about extreme things that can frighten both therapists and family members present. They might talk about the voices telling them to kill. Similarly, one might talk about frightening visual sensations. Strong paranoid belief systems can also put therapists in challenging situations when the person gives detailed evidence of events in their life to justify the beliefs. The person may demand an answer as to whether others share their beliefs. In a crisis, arguing about the reality of a help-seeker's experiences does not open the door to dialogue and a multi-dimensional examination of one's own life. What matters most is to focus on the emotional experiences of the person in need of help, for example, when they tell us about the persecutors who are following them. This can be done in a simple way, for example by saying "that situation must feel really hard for you" or "I understand that this has been very difficult for you—could you tell me how you feel when you are threatened?" Such comments can help open space for broader reflection on life, including aspects that are not related to threatening psychotic experiences.

Attention Primarily on the Presence Here and Now

In dialogical practice, this is one of the most important guidelines for action. Instead of focusing primarily on the life events that clients tell us about, we focus more on what happens when they talk about their experiences, and how the responses to what they say reciprocally affect the experiences of the participants in the conversation. Anything that has happened prior to this conversation can be discussed, focusing on the main emotions that arise when talking. The actual event is, in a sense, secondary in that talking about the situation may lead us to share the most relevant emotional experiences. In psychotic crises, there are additional elements that underline the importance of this approach. While one with psychotic experience may be talking about something that we as clinicians might consider psychotic experiences, they may be talking for the first time about extreme experiences in their lives for which they have had no words.

An important observation is that, at the beginning of a crisis, the window is often open to the sensations experienced by the person in need of help and they are willing to talk about them. For example, someone may be ready to talk about "strange thoughts" when in a strong emotional state. When the situation calms down, he is no longer interested in talking about these potentially frightening experiences. It is then important that we, as clinicians, are awake and seize the moment when the person who needs help starts to talk about, for example, "strange thoughts." It is at that moment that they come into contact with their own most difficult experiences, which have no other way of being expressed than, for example, through hallucinations. I always pay attention to this, even if it means interrupting an ongoing conversation. As the study comparing good and bad treatment outcomes points out (see Chap. 9), the opportunity to talk about psychotic experiences may be lost altogether if not encouraged in the moment.

The Open Dialogue approach has proven highly effective in supporting people with psychosis to return to active working life. In fact, the actual clinical practice—how therapists talk with those having psychotic experiences—appears broadly similar across a range of effective psychotherapeutic methods. In cognitive behavioral therapy, too, one of the basic principles is the normalization of psychotic experience (Freeman & Garety, 2006). Similar to what I have described in this chapter, Freeman and Garety say that "paranoid ideation is an appropriate strategy that can, under certain circumstances, become overwhelming, just as in intense anxiety" (p. 407).

References

Abettan, C. (2015). The current dialogue between phenomenology and psychiatry: A problematic misunderstanding. *Medical Health Care and Philosophy, 18*(4), 533–540.

Avdi, E., Lerou, V., & Seikkula, J. (2015). Dialogical features, therapist responsiveness, and agency in a therapy for psychosis. *Journal of Constructivist Psychology, 28*(4), 329–341.

Carman, T. (2008). *Merleau-Ponty*. Routledge. https://doi.org/10.4324/9780203461853

De Leede-Smith, S., & Barkus, E. (2014). A comprehensive review of auditory verbal hallucinations: Lifetime prevalence, correlates and mechanisms in healthy and clinical individuals. *Frontiers in Human Neuroscience*. Current perspectives on the mechanisms of auditory hallucinations in clinical and non-clinical populations, 62–86.

Freeman, D., & Garety, P. (2006). Helping patients with paranoid and suspicious thoughts: A cognitive-behavioural approach. *Adverse Psychiatric Treatment, 2*(6), 404–415.

Haarakangas, K. (1997). *Voices of the treatment meeting* (p. 130). Jyväskylä Studies in Education, Psychology and Social Research.

Holma, J., & Aaltonen, J. (1997). The sense of agency and the search for a narrative in acute psychosis. *Contemporary Family Therapy, 19*(4), 463–477.

Karon, B. P. (2003). The tragedy of schizophrenia without psychotherapy. *Journal of American Academy of Psychoanalysis and Dynamic Psychiatry, 31*(1), 89–118.
Karon, B., & Vandenbos, G. (1981). *Psychotherapy of schizophrenia. The treatment of choice*. Jason Aronson.
Levinas, I. (1985). *Ethics and infinity*. Duquesne University Press.
Lysaker, P., & Lysaker, J. (2004). Dialogical transformation in the psychotherapy of schizophrenia. In H. Hermans & C. Dimaggio (Eds.), *The dialogical self in psychotherapy* (pp. 205–219). Brunner/Routledge.
Mitropoulos, G. (2020). Auditory verbal hallucinations in psychosis abnormal perceptions or symptoms of disordered thought? *The Journal of Nervous and Mental Disease, 208*(1).
Moncrieff, J., & Leo, J. (2010). A systematic review of the effects of antipsychotic drugs on brain volume. *Psychological Medicine, 40*(9), 1409–1422. https://doi.org/10.1017/S0033291709992297
Read, J., Goodman, L., Morrison, A., Ross, C., & Aderhold, V. (2004). Childhood trauma, loss and stress. In J. Read, L. Mosher, & R. B. Ventall (Eds.), *Models of madness* (pp. 223–253). Brunner-Routledge. https://doi.org/10.4324/9780203420393_chapter_16
Roe, D., & Davidson, L. (2005). Self and narrative in schizophrenia: Time to author a new story. *Medical Humanities, 31*(2), 89–94.
Trimble, D. (2000). Emotion and voice in network therapy. *Netletter, 7*(1), 11–16.
van der Kolk, B. A., McFarlane, A. C., & Weisaeth, L. (Eds.). (2006). *Traumatic stress*. Guilford.

Chapter 8
Dialogue Develops Reflexivity

The dialogical orientation has created ways of determining the quality of the dialogue and improving it. Healing dialogues can be explored to find the best ways to help others and develop self-reflective dialogue. In a dialogical experience, life management is improved through increased reflexivity. By increasing their opportunities to reflect on their own feelings and experiences, clients can gain greater control over their life's dilemmas and resources to cope with difficult crises. At its best, this growth in reflection can mean that people take more responsibility for their own affairs and, consequently, for the factors that influence the crisis. This increase in reflexivity and its dialogical promotion will be discussed in this chapter.

Experiencing Emotions Diversifies Life

A friend of mine told me a story about her brother. She told me that the rest of the family was quite worried about him because he didn't share his feelings much and didn't seem to be very involved in his new family life. The brother and his wife had two children: a 7-year-old daughter and an 8-year-old son.

Six months earlier, after 3 years abroad, the brother and his family moved back home. As their financial situation was very poor and they needed a new start in life urgently, my friend offered the brother's family the opportunity to live with her in her house, as her older children had already moved out on their own. The youngest daughter was still in high school.

Living with his sister seemed to be very distressing for her brother. Life was run by his wife, who took care of all practical matters. He did drive the car to the supermarket and did what he was told, but he did not take an active part in the upbringing of the household or the children. His wife had already started talking to my friend, saying that she might not want to continue together because she felt she had three children to look after.

J. Seikkula, *Why Dialogue Does Cure*,
https://doi.org/10.1007/978-3-031-91294-8_8

Life with two small and lively children was very noisy, and gradually they took over the main part of my friend's home, which began to distress her daughter and herself. She had already got used to the quiet, low-noise rhythm of life and now it seemed that there was hardly ever a chance to relax and enjoy the quiet. It was also impossible to invite friends over, as the house was no longer her territory.

After 6 months, the brother's family was offered a house to rent where they could live for at least a year. The house was very nice, in its own peace and quiet, with a small yard. When they went to visit it, both the brother's wife and the children immediately fell in love with it. The brother, on the other hand, was afraid because it would be a big financial responsibility in a situation where both of their jobs were precarious. But his wife pressed him, saying that she would move in on her own, and he could return to his mother if he did not want to follow them.

The brother was forced to move, and they did so within a couple of weeks. That same weekend, some of the family had gathered for a communal lunch. They expected the brother's family to be there, too. The brother arrived before his wife and children. My friend told me that everyone had been excited to hear what they thought of the new home. In particular, many asked what the children thought of the new home. The air was full of questions for a brother who was not used to talking and reflecting.

He tried to cope by saying that the children liked their new home. How, tell me, how do they like it? What did they say? Did they play there? How did all this play out? Interested questions poured in. The brother who was anxious about the questions replied that he couldn't say or describe it better than, "It sounds like you have a lot of questions, and I can't pinpoint all those children's feelings. I am like that," said the brother. To my friend's surprise, she had seen a tear in the corner of her brother's eye.

Reflection Opens Up New Opportunities

Something new and revolutionary happened at that very moment when the family bombarded the brother with questions. The brother, after what had obviously been a very pleasant experience, became moved to tell about how much the children had liked their new home. At the same time, he said something unexpected: He described to the others how he *felt about* their questions, how he *saw himself in relation to them,* how he *recognized that he* could not answer them, and how he *reflected that* that was the kind of man he was. Perhaps maybe even for the very first time in his life, he did something we can use the word "reflect" to describe. This was most probably aided by his emotion at that moment when he said something so enormous to those close to him. My friend told me that she was speechless because she had never heard her brother say anything like that before.

This is what we can aim for in dialogical practices. Canadian psychotherapist Lynn Agnus describes how clients in psychotherapy talk about their issues—including their feelings—on three different levels. The first level is external language, where we talk about things by describing something that is happening. Often in this kind of description, we are an outside observer of events. For example, at the beginning of therapy, clients use a lot of this language to describe their lives and why they sought therapy. The second, already slightly more developed level, is internal language. Here people also describe their own inner experiences. For example, they talk about how they were scared or how they got angry or how they became happy. And then there is the third level, reflective language, where people reflect on their inner experience in relation to their relationships and their own experiences. It was this huge leap that I heard my friend's brother do as he took in that emotional moment with his relatives.

In Chap. 5, I already described some of Tom Andersen's pioneering work. Tom often talked about the emergence of inner reflection as the goal of psychotherapy. How can we promote reflection in the dialogues to help people who need help take control of their own lives? What kind of dialogue-facilitator skills are needed in crisis situations to generate reflective dialogues?

Dialogue Creates Resources

Studies of Open Dialogue have provided ample evidence that dialogical practice can generate unprecedented resources in difficult crises. However, we have not had enough information on what kind of dialogues with people in need are worth having to increase their resources. This is a question that I have tried to address in several research projects.

I first became interested in the subject when we started to get unexpectedly good results in the treatment of psychotic crises in Western Lapland. All along, I have understood that the best results come from the overall treatment and the integration of the important treatment factors. Within this framework, I created the first research project in the early 2000s to investigate the differences between the dialogues of therapy meetings in treatment processes that led to good treatment outcomes and poor treatment outcomes (Seikkula, 2002). I selected patients treated in two research cohorts of psychosis patients between 1992 and 1997 as subjects for evaluation. I selected ten treatment processes with poor treatment outcomes for review. In these, after 2 years, the patient still had psychotic problems affecting his/her life or was on sick leave or disability pension. For these 10, I chose pairs of controls in which the initial treatment situation had been similar, but the treatment outcome had been good. They were in employment and no longer had psychotic problems.

I examined the first therapy meetings of all processes by analyzing the dialogue. To understand the meaningful features of the dialogue, I discovered the IR (Initiative—Response Analysis) method developed by Linell (1998) from Sweden. In the analysis, his research team was interested in who dominated the dialogue in three different formats. *Quantitative dominance* refers to who speaks the most on each topic. *Semantic dominance* describes who takes the initiative and determines the topic of the discussion. *Interactional dominance* describes how people talk. A simple example of interactional dominance is when the therapist asks the client, "What do you think about this issue, Dad?" In this way, the therapist determines who will participate in the conversation next. Interaction dominance is also the case for the person who starts crying and whose crying silences the other person's speech.

In addition to these dominant features, I was interested in whether the conversation was monologic or dialogical. In a monologic conversation, for example, we ask questions to which there is a right answer. We are asking for information about something, clarifying something, or making a decision. Monological discussions are also debates, where no one gives up their position because they think it is the only correct one. Dialogue, on the other hand, is where each person puts forward their own point of view and expects the other to add their own. All expressions are open to receive the other's comment and are not completed until the other responds. And the other's response usually opens up another invitation to complete what has been said. It is the dialogue itself, not the participants in the conversation, that begins to guide the course of the discussion. This kind of dialogical dialogue was originally discussed by Luckman (1990). These moments of dialogical dialogue can easily be seen in the therapy meeting described in Chap. 2.

In the research projects on psychosis, our attention had been drawn to some families with whom it seemed very difficult to establish any kind of reflective space. We noticed that these therapy meetings were talking about practical issues and phenomena, but not really reflecting on the inner experiences of the participants. In the 1930s, the Russian psychologist Lev Vygotsky drew attention to a stage in the development of human language, which he called indicative language. This stage of development is before a child develops symbolic language around the age of 12. I think that the way these families spoke was very similar to this. When you talk about a phenomenon, there has to be a physical counterpart. The language was very concrete and indicative. It is possible that a difficult crisis can concretize our language in this way, reducing our ability to reflect on the different dimensions of things.

The purpose of a dialogue analysis is to look at a conversation from beginning to end and see how it develops. According to Linell's method, a conversation is divided into topical episodes that define what is discussed about. In this study, there were roughly 30 such topical episodes in one therapy meeting of about 1.5 h. Table 8.1 summarizes the dialogues from the first 10 treatment meetings with good treatment outcomes and the first 10 meetings with poor treatment outcomes.

Table 8.1 Differences between the dialogues in the topical episodes of good and poor treatment outcomes

	Good treatment result	Poor treatment result
Clients' interaction dominance	**55–57%**	**10–35%**
Clients' semantic dominance	**70%**	**40–70%**
Symbolic language area in the topical episodes	**67–80%**	**0–20%**
Dialogical dialogue in the topical episodes	**60–65%**	**10–50%**

Percentage of all topical episodes. Statistically significant difference in bold

One of my first observations was that the *quantitative dominance* of the discussion did not play much of a role in describing the nature of the therapy meeting. The semantic dominance of clients also did not distinguish between good and poor outcomes. In contrast, there was a significant difference in the dominance of interactional dominance of the conversation. In the good treatment outcomes, in more than half of all topical episodes, clients had interactional dominance compared to only less than a third in the poor treatment outcomes. This reflects the fact that in well-performing treatments, clients largely determined how the dialogue proceeded. For example, by changing their own emotional state, they could influence the rhythm and other aspects of the conversation. Similarly, very clear differences emerged in terms of symbolic language and dialogical dialogue. In the well-performing treatments, most conversations took place in the symbolic language domain. In the poor ones, the situation was reversed: more than 80% of the topical episodes took place by speaking in indicative, concrete terms. Dialogical dialogues were characteristic of well-performing treatments, whereas they were rarely used in poorly performing treatments.

I have described these results on several occasions before, and there is no need to repeat what has been said before. However, to summarize this study, it is important to highlight a few points:

1) The construction of a symbolic language of meaning paves the way for change so that clients' agency increases and symptoms decrease. This is not up to the therapy team alone, but it is important to learn skills to facilitate reflective comments. As noted in Chap. 6, dialogical and reflective change does not occur at the moment of clients' autonomic nervous system arousal, but afterward. This skill requires therapists to be particularly sensitive to when it is appropriate to ask reflective questions of clients; for example, "What meaning do you give to this feeling?" or, "What are all the thoughts that this sad experience of yours evokes?" Therefore, it is good to live with strong emotions as they occur and to ask reflective questions and comments afterward.

A particular challenge for clinicians is posed by conversations that take place in the indicative meaning domain of the language. In these cases, most of the attention seems to go to describing and discussing concrete events, rather than reflecting on them. In some cases, the team may try to generate reflection among themselves, but if the team is talking in the symbolic domain, it will not resonate with the family, who at that moment are thinking about everything in concrete terms. In one treatment process, we watched the recordings of the therapy meeting in the research group and drew attention to the painful experience of the team when nothing seemed to resonate. Change began to occur when we suggested that it was indeed worthwhile for the team to have a reflective discussion with each other. However, in that discussion, one could only refer to things that everyone could see or otherwise identify. It is very important to introduce statements by saying, for example, "What my mother said about my father not being involved in the family's joint decisions made me think of......" Or: "When Risto talked about his mother and touched her, I remembered that....." In that particular case, which was of concern to our research team, the first sign of change was that the young mother, suffering from depression, started to become very angry, and in a frenzy of anger started to speak on a metaphorical level. "I'm sick and tired of everyone talking s***." Now these very harsh outbursts were metaphorical, because the feces in question were not visible, but were just a phrase and metaphor that had come to the mind of the client. The raw emotion of the experience opened the way to slowly begin to build a space for symbolic language. Interestingly, this family began to talk about childhood fairy tales and their meaning for both the young mother of the family and her mother.

2) The creation of dialogue opens the way to a common shared emotional experience and thus to an increased ability to tolerate the uncertainty of the crisis and to start talking about the most difficult issues. The therapy meeting we presented in Chap. 2 provides many examples of this. For example, when the mother at the very beginning of the discussion said she wanted to talk about what she had done wrong as a mother:

Jaakko: Yes, I hear you saying that you want to get an answer to what happened when your daughter had similar problems.

Helena: Yes, because as a mother you ask what I did wrong. Even though you were doing your best, you failed. Do you understand? Liisa didn't want to... she lost the will to live because she had a little boy who was a normal child until he was three and a half, so to speak. Now he's a 13-year-old special child. He doesn't walk, he doesn't talk, he doesn't hear anymore. He is totally dependent on his mother. Liisa gave up her own life to live her child's life today. As for Natalia, I don't know what happened. Now she has succeeded in her life and her profession. Sometimes I ask myself what I did wrong.

Jaakko: Yes, I heard you say that you think to yourself what you did wrong. How did you fail?

Helena: Yes, because as a mother I feel like a failure. Why did this happen to my daughters? (Moves and tears).

((8))

Jaakko: I hear you say that as a mother I failed...

Helena: Yes, for me...

Jaakko: When I hear what you say, I get a little sad. When I feel sad, I often feel it here (strokes his upper stomach with his hand). Now I feel a little sad.

Helena: That's how I feel.

In this conversation, a shared emotional experience is immediately shared, from the fact that the mother's message was very emotional to the therapist's courageous acceptance of the mother's message and her reference to her own physical experience of feeling a little sad in his stomach. Such periods of discussion, when participants feel something "vibrating within themselves" (the expression of one of my colleagues) are indeed important moments. *The skill required of therapists is to hear what clients are saying and to follow it unconditionally, without imposing it as a guideline for their own therapeutic work.* What seems to be particularly important is that therapists do not set out to make some therapeutic intervention but share the situation as it arises.

An example of this was a family discussion in which a colleague had invited me to broaden his perspective on a family problem. The parents were very angry and worried about their 19-year-old son, who for the last year or so had stopped wanting to take part in anything the family did together and was just rejecting his parents and saying he wasn't interested. The parents also felt that he was very passive-aggressive towards them. This conversation was the first one with all three of them together and my colleague had met with each of them alone before.

In particular, the father talked a lot about his disappointment that their son was not taking on adult responsibilities. The mother and son sat side by side and the mother often told her son what the father said and might even stroke his back when he said it. When my colleague and I had a reflective conversation with each other, my colleague said that she had drawn attention to the fact that the mother was acting as an intermediary between father and son. She went on to say that a change was needed whereby the mother could relinquish this role. I was a little startled by this blunt strategic aim and asked her to help me make sure I understood what she meant. She confirmed that this was exactly what she wanted. To this, I replied that I was surprised by her observation. It sounds interesting because I had thought of another aspect of that phenomenon, I said. I felt it was important that at least two members of the family could still communicate with each other, especially when father and son are at a breaking point.

With this comment, I did not want to challenge my colleague's comment, but I did want to slow down the momentum so that we do not go straight to the strategic effort to change the triangle of the family system. I can't say it's a better course of action than the other, but this example illustrates how in a dialogical conversation, we seek to build a shared experience, not make a change in the family. After we as the therapy team started to reflect on the different meanings of the performance, the son started to participate more in the conversation with his comments.

Another important finding from my research is related to understanding the importance of dialogical dialogue. It turned out that about one-third of the topical episodes in well-done treatments could also be monologic. It is therefore important to accept those topical episodes in which, for example, information is shared, questions are answered, treatment agreements are made, and things are clarified, as an important part of the dialogical work. The division between monologue being bad and dialogue being good is not the basis of dialogical practice, but both forms of communication are needed for a good encounter. The facilitators need to learn skills for a specific response in every moment of the conversation to adapt to the specific needs of the conversation. Sometimes really it is advisable to give direct answers to direct questions.

We can take a look at an example of a therapy meeting, which was referred to earlier in Chap. 7. It is an example of dialogue that did not lead to a good outcome. In this passage, Pekka (name changed) describes the events that led to his admission to the hospital. I have often used this example to describe what happens when the team does not respond to the patient's initial reflection on their own actions. But beyond that, it reflects an indicative language and the fact that in this passage the person is not reaching for a symbolic meaning.

On Monday morning, the team (T1 is the ward psychiatrist, T2 is the nurse who met Pekka and his family on a home visit the previous week) meets Pekka (P) and during the conversation, it is revealed that the reason for the hospital admission is that Pekka has been violent at home.

T1: I think it happened in the last 2 weeks, not before.

T2: Was it just a threat, or worse?

T1: Hitting, I think Pekka has hit his mother.

(...)

T1: I understood that Pekka had tried to ask his mother something.

P: Well, it was last weekend when the police came to our house. He was drunk. When he didn't say anything and started making coffee even though it was the middle of the night. And I asked... I went out and came into the kitchen and he turned around and told me not to talk about it. And then I just slapped her. He ran out into the hallway and started screaming. And I said there's no need to shout, why can't she tell me? And then I started to calm down... and that's when the feeling came... and that's when the police came. But somehow I feel that no, of course, it's not allowed to hit anyone. But there are situations that...

T1: When did you go to the health center?

P: Yeah, this happened just before that.

T1: Why didn't the mother say the police came?

P: What?

T2: Why didn't it say that the police were at your house last night?

P: It wasn't last night, it was last weekend. I was thinking, I keep thinking about all these weird things and I knew they weren't true. But when you think about them for a while you get the feeling that something like that could have really happened... It's just too... you just think about weird things.

T2: And this all started last weekend, this situation?

T1: Yes.

Pekka described the events very concretely and in detail, even repeating the dialogue between him and his mother before he "slapped" her. It seems significant that at the end of his description, he begins to reflect on the justification of his actions. Unfortunately, the team is so interested in what happened at home that they do not hear Pekka's reflection, nor do they respond to it, but continue to question him about what happened. In the next contribution, Pekka still reflects on the strange thoughts (i.e., talks about his psychotic experiences), which sometimes he could distinguish as untrue, but sometimes not. A window opened to start talking about these inner experiences, but the team continued to explore what happened at home and missed the opportunity to start reflecting.

It may be that the concreteness of the language spoken makes it difficult to be sensitive to Pekka's reflections on his own violence and his own psychotic experiences. It is thoughtful to note that Pekka himself took the initiative and opened a window for this reflection, but when the team did not take it up, never later in Pekka's treatment did it become possible to talk about his psychotic experiences. Violence was discussed afterward.

Dialogue Is the Art of Responding

This method of exploring dialogue was further developed a few years later in a project exploring couples therapy for depressed people, particularly its dialogical and narrative dimensions (Seikkula et al., 2011). With our research team, we became more interested in the possibility of understanding the nature of a multidisciplinary dialogue—two clients and two therapists. To this end, we developed the Dialogical Investigations for Happening of Change (DIHC) method with Belgian family therapist and professor Peter Rober and professor Aarno Laitila. We added to the first version of the research method a special focus on the recording of response habits. In addition to the previous variables, we were also interested in what is answered and not answered in the expressions and how the response is made. The way of responding is described both by verbal expressions, for example, whether the narrative is dialogical or monologic, and by how we respond with body movements, voice inflections, glances, and other non-verbal ways. We were also more interested in the importance of being present in the here-and-now as observed in the above example. We asked whether we were responding to something that had happened before, or to a previous moment of conversation, for example, or to what was happening in the present moment.

DIHC Method for Assessing the Quality of Dialogue

To clarify the dialogue, the therapy conversations must be recorded. After the recording, the conversation of the session can be transcribed into a text. Each session is then divided into topical episodes. The topical episode is defined according to the subject being discussed. The same topic can therefore be discussed more than once. Each topical episode is then evaluated by each of the variables I will describe below. This type of analysis can be used, for example, to understand what happened in your own therapy sessions. In a scientific study, it is useful to write down the statements of each speaker in a separate column, so that it is easy to see each speaker's contribution to the dialogue.

The actual analysis is done in stages.

STEP 1: Identifying topical episodes.

The following variables will be assessed for each topical episode.

STEP II: How to respond.

A response is not a direct comment on a single expression, but an evolving event, possibly involving several contributions and comments. It is important to note the three stages of the dialogical process. First, there is the expression/utterance—which of course is often already a response to some utterance that preceded it—and the response of the listener to that expression. The meaning of the response can only be understood from the comment of the original speaker to the comment of the interlocutor. From this sequence of events, we can then determine more precisely who dominates this specific topical episode and in what way.

The main interest is not so much the determination of dominance, but more about being in line with the nature of therapeutic dialogue, how initiatives change during the course of the discussion.

The next step is to find out what the response is. Very rarely—if ever—does a response answer everything that is said. The respondent always chooses what to answer. He or she may respond to something the speaker says, choosing one theme, he or she may respond to an emotional state conveyed by the speaker, and he or she may respond to something already said. The respondent can also respond to something expressed that has happened outside the session or, for example, in a previous therapy session. What is most interesting is to see how the response affects the flow of the dialogue.

It is at least as interesting to find out what is not answered. We can never answer everything, and it is not even a meaningful endeavor. In our response, we always choose something, and the choices we make affect the course of the dialogue. Fortunately for us, in a dialogical encounter, there is no one right answer and therefore no one right way to proceed, but several different paths that develop the dialogical process. However, there are also answers that end the dialogue, as we saw in the example above.

The next question is how we respond. Answers can be monological answers to monological questions. For example, conveying information about a topic, where the elucidation of that information is an important monologic conversation. The response can also be one that generates a dialogue. That is dialogical dialogue, to use Luckmann's term. In a dialogical response, the speaker always incorporates the preceding utterance into his own following utterance. The subject is not completed without taking into account the response of the other.

This way of responding also includes the question of how we consider what is happening here-and-now in our response and create a shared emotional experience. How do we manage to be present for the participants in the conversation at the very moment when the opportunity opens up to confront something essential that has not yet been said?

STEP III: Determining the language and/or narrative process of the meeting.

There are two different ways to do this. First, it can be used to determine whether the language domain of the conversation is indicative or symbolic (Vygotsky, 1935; Haarakangas, 1997; Wertsch, 1991). Each topical episode in the discussion is defined as one or the other.

As a second option, the language domain of the conversation can also be explored using a special Narrative Process Coding System developed by Angus et al. (1999). This concept was further developed by Aarno Laitila for application in family and couple's therapy. In line with Angus' original assumption, for example, in individual psychotherapy, the proportion of reflective speech increases as the therapy progresses.

After analyzing each topical episode using these variables, an overall picture emerges of how the dialogue progresses from one topic to the next. Based on this overview, we can select specific topical episodes for closer micro-analysis, allowing us, for example, to identify the points at which a dialogical shift began to take place.

Together with Mary Olson, we wrote a chapter in the book Research Methods in Couples Therapy (Seikkula & Olson, 2016). In it, we analyzed one couples therapy process in more detail. This example illustrates well how we divide a therapy session into topical episodes and how in each topical episode we scrutinize all the dialogical variables described above. When we combine the results of these topical episodes, we get an accurate description of the nature of the dialogue and at which point the dialogical change occurs.

In this particular therapy session, Victoria and Alfonso had a total of four sessions, three of which were specifically about their problems, and the final session was about how they had solved their problems during the three sessions. The first three sessions covered 20, 21, and 20 topical episodes respectively (Table 8.2). In the first session, both therapists and Victoria took a lot of initiative in terms of topics of discussion (semantic dominance) and interaction (interaction dominance). Alfonso took the initiative in only three topical episodes in the session. In the second meeting, there was a turnaround in that Alfonso became much more active and this continued in the third session. It can also be seen that the number of dialogical topical episodes increased significantly in the third session. Based on this simple classification, attention turns to the second discussion: What in particular happened so that Alfonso became much more active and how did this all contribute to the fact that there was much more dialogical sharing in the subsequent discussion than before?

Table 8.2 Summary of the categories of topical episodes in the three therapy sessions with Victoria and Alfonso

		Semantic dominance	Interactional dominance	Monologue s. dialogue	Indicative vs. symbolic
First session	*Victoria*	14	9		
	Alfonso	3	0		
	Therapists	3	11		
	Total	20	20	16 vs. 4	14 vs. 6
Second session	*Victoria*	8	5		
	Alfonso	6	5		
	Therapists	7	11		
	Total	21	21	12 vs. 9	13 vs. 8
Third session	*Victoria*	6	6		
	Alfonso	5	2		
	Therapists	9	12		
	Total	20	20	9 vs. 11	8 vs. 12

Sharing for Dialogue

The start of the second session felt rather chaotic and tense. Therapist 1 saw Victoria and Alfonso coming into the building for the consultation. The couple seemed very agitated, and Alfonso had to encourage Victoria to come into the office.

At the beginning of the session, the therapist asked how they felt today. Alfonso said, "pretty good." Victoria replied that she felt differently and did not want to come to the session. She said she was tired. From a dialogical perspective, her expression "I am tired" and saying that she did not want to come to the session may have reflected a lack of dialogical context, in that there was no common language in which she could describe and share her feelings. Her comment was monological in the sense that she was simply stating the state of affairs without giving space to the listener's comments.

Victoria began to talk about her and Alfonso's relationship with disappointment. Twice she said she was sad. The last time, the therapists had given them a homework assignment to set aside some time each evening for a joint conversation. Victoria was disappointed with this task because Alfonso had been away so many nights that they hadn't done the task.

Alfonso tried to explain his part, but his speech was so garbled that it was difficult to get his message across. He started sentences that he never finished. Both spoke in monologues, expressing their own thoughts without any attempt at sharing.

Victoria said she was depressed and tired of her job. She said, "I've been working about 15 hours every day and I'm never home. And then when I come back in the evening, he's not there because he's meeting some friends..."

The therapist replied:

T1: You said "never." What does that mean?

A: That I am never at home

T1: Now that you said you are never at home, you are never at home together?

This simple repetition of Victoria's statement seemed to change the communication so that Victoria began to talk more concretely about her concerns. This comment by the therapist seemed to contribute towards dialogical communication though it seemed challenging. The therapist's comment on this single word also seemed to communicate that she was present to actively listen to them and at the same time to seek other meanings for Victoria's concerns.

After this short period of discussion, the conversation became more interactive. Victoria was no longer alone with her own tiredness and sadness. Alfonso also began to express himself more clearly and precisely. The therapist's simple and minimal commentary seemed to help create a dialogical interaction, addressing shared concerns rather than the separate and disconnected concerns of each.

From Dialogue to Reflection

Then, after about 5 min, the therapist asked them how they would like to use the time. They both wanted to talk about Alfonso's upcoming trip home. This topic is very important and even traumatic for Victoria. Two years earlier they had travelled together to meet Alfonso's parents and Victoria had actively tried to make friends with Alfonso's mother, but she had refused to say a word to Victoria. For Victoria, the experience was terrible, and after this trip, she became depressed and was on sick leave for a year. Understandably, therefore, this was a very tense subject for both spouses.

In what follows, I will present two different topical episodes that illustrate in particular the emergence of Alfonso's reflection in the second episode. In the first episode, his expressions are so fragmented that it is difficult to make out what he is saying.

In the Beginning There Was Great Confusion

The discussion starts with Alfonso describing what he has planned to do at home. Victoria responds aggressively and Alfonso starts to defend himself. The beginning of the conversation was monologue-like in that both told their own point of view to each other without sharing. The beginning of the conversation sequence was not changed even by the therapist's comments and questions about their emotional experiences.

In Table 8.3, I will present the conversation between Victoria and Alfonso, following the research methodology of the DIHC method. All speakers have their own columns so that you can see the topic of each speaker and what was said. The first snippet starts after 16 minutes since the beginning of the session. Alfonso speaks a lot but in a very unclear way. This may reflect his lack of words for his experience, or, on the other hand, he is trying to balance himself so as not to provoke a negative response from Victoria.

In this episode, Alfonso talks a lot. He does not express complete sentences, but fragmented thoughts. These are different voices, but these voices are not polyphonic in such a way that they would form a coherent story or its beginning. Victoria listens and seems to reach for something of what Alfonso is trying to say, and in another sequence of the conversations, begins to talk about her own feelings, fear, and abandonment. At first, it seems that Alfonso is not affected by this.

Table 8.3 New topical episode: Alfonson's visit to his family

Victoria	Alfonso	Therapists	Classification
	Well, I'm going to visit home for a week's trip.		A semantic dominance
		Hmh	
	I think it would be good to see... For example, the last time I went home, these things.... That you want to get WhatsApp. Now is a good time to practice...		Voices: Previous visit to a's home Address to Victoria
		What do you think about it, the visit?	Answer: Visit Not answered: Uncertainty
	(7) I'd like to think that there might be days when...It might happen that I can't... Although it was said that I could communicate... Then on the other hand...		Answered: Victoria Voices: People at home
What can't you do? Send me a WhatsApp			Interactional dominance Positioning: Aggressive, wants contact
	I just said I could send it. And I'm there for like a week, even if I call, maybe I can or maybe I can't, I'm very busy... I can do this, I can send WhatsApp, but if one time happens or I can't put a message right away... Like, if you could try to understand that that could happen...		Voices: People at home Positioning: Lower, asking for understanding and defending his actions
Yes, I can try. I think it's just such an easy thing to do if you want to			Answered: Alfonso and the dilemma he experienced at home Opening dialogue

(continued)

Table 8.3 (continued)

Victoria	Alfonso	Therapists	Classification
	Yes, but I can tell you that sometimes it can happen that if somehow I can call you in the evening, then sometimes it can happen, but that...If I have a lot of different things to do there, then it can happen that if we call in the evening...		Voices: People at home Address: The voices of home Monolog
Yes, of course, we can't call every night			Positioning: Not any more offensive
	Why not?		
Because it has always happened. I don't even need, I don't even need....			Positioning: Felt like menacing
	Okay (7)		
New topical episode	***Victoria's***	***Fear***	
		And what do you think about this?	Interactional dominance
[well, I'm scared because]		Alfonso, visiting his home?	
Now it has been there three times alone and each time I have been very sad. Sometimes I feel like he doesn't really have time to WhatsApp me, how can it really be like that? I have the feeling that I am nothing to him when he is there at home... Sometimes			Voices: Previous visits Positioning: Weak and powerless Address: Alfonso and his brother-in-law
		Hmhm	
But I've felt this way every time at some point			
		So... You have known?	Answered: Emotional experience
That he doesn't think about me and wants to forget me when he's there			Positioning: Weaker than Alfonso's family

(continued)

Table 8.3 (continued)

Victoria	Alfonso	Therapists	Classification
		And what does it mean that you feel he wants to forget you? (points with hand in the direction of Alfonso)	Answered: Here-and-now In the form of a question
I feel like, I don't know... It doesn't seem possible, how Alfonso can be so busy that he doesn't have time to think about me and write a message... That sometimes I just don't get it. You don't have to call me. I just need to know that you're thinking about me			Voices: Abandoned Positioning: Between Alfonso and his brother-in-law Asking to choose
	But I've never felt that way without messaging you at least once a day		Not answered: Victoria's feeling

Alfonso Begins to Speak Reflectively

Later on, the same topic will be discussed on a more general level. In this episode, several dialogical connections are established, and Alfonso speaks clearly, referring to himself as an actor. In this episode, Alfonso begins to reflectively consider his role after the therapists actively seek to clarify what he meant. The conversation presented in Table 8.4 takes place after 42 min.

At the beginning of the topical episode, the therapist repeats word for word what Alfonso said and asks for further clarification. Alfonso replies to the therapist, which is apparently easier than addressing Victoria directly. But of course, Victoria is involved in this conversation by listening and addressing Alfonso as one of the addressees about what she has said. At least it seems that way, because Alfonso's statements are clearer than before. The sentences have a clear subject, "I," and the stories told include a beginning, middle, and end. The therapist's summation that all this seems to have become a big deal in their relationship is confirmed by both of them. It seems that the therapist asked this reflective question at just the right moment after the emotional turmoil. After this, Victoria is no longer on the offensive, but surprisingly protects Alfonso by saying that she does not want him to come between the two families. This comment is followed by a dialogue that further defines the relationship between Victoria, Alfonso, and his family.

The style of the dialogue that started here continued until the end of the session. The reflection was dialogical, both speaking in the first-person form, pointing words

Table 8.4 Alfonso begins to speak reflectively

Victoria	Alfonso	Therapists	Categories
	I just think that every time we've been somewhere together, I'm there and you're not. When I'm there, for you it's... It's not normal time on a normal day, it's...		Semantic dominance Positioning: Defensive Monologue
		I didn't quite understand what you meant, Alfonso, that every time you're apart, you're...	Dialogue Trying to intervene in a dialogical way
	Whenever I've been home though, when Victoria is here		
		Okay	
	... So it's a different day for me	[it is therefore not the same]	
	Yes, it's not the same situation, we're in two different places. It's... We're apart, like in a different context		Alfonso finds more words to reflect on the experience
		This seems to have become a big thing in your relationship. Lots of details about your relationship	Try to find a way to talk in concrete terms like Victoria and about events like Alfonso
Yes. It's a big deal. And I know that family is important and I've tried... I don't want Alfonso to be between two families...			Answered: Alfonso Address: Therapist and Alfonso Dialogue Understand more about their place
	Hmh	Hmh	
...But I've tried. Sometimes I wonder if they're deliberately trying to keep you so busy that you don't have time for me. Because it's obvious they don't like me			For the first time, the silenced voice is out in the open: The family members of Alfonso don't like Victoria

(continued)

Table 8.4 (continued)

Victoria	Alfonso	Therapists	Categories
		What is the situation?	Dialogue
That he must be between two fires			
		I see... You think Alfonso's family wants him to be in between	Dialogue Here-and-now
Yes, it seems that way. I've been trying to...			Dialogue
	Yes. There's also the thing that I don't care what my family wants to say to me. Or if they don't want to come visit me here, it's really not important. If it was just me		Answered: The concern of Victoria Positioning: Defensive Address: Alfonso's family
		Okay	
	And what she says is that it's important to them	[yhmm]	
	...My life here, they would come and visit me		
I don't think it's fair to Alfonso that he has to be in a situation where there are two different families and he has to sort of... That he has to travel all the time			Answered: Alfonso's situation Here-and-now Dialogue Understanding
	It's not a big deal for me, because when I go home, I also meet my friends		Dialogue Voices of friends Not so a loaded subject
		Hmhh	

at each other. They also clarified each other and raised contradictions. A dialogue developed between them. They had more than 20 exchanges without a single comment from the therapists. Alfonso remembered one phone call he had made to Victoria on his way home from work. Victoria said it made her happy.

The second period of conversation described above contains the part where the change in the second session took place in the way that reflection began. Victoria and Alfonso spoke to each other in a different way than at the beginning of the session. The therapists were actively involved in the discussion with short repetitions of what was said or with specific questions. They did not open any new topic, but their comments were systematic comments on the themes opened by the clients. The therapists also accepted their new role as listeners to Alfonso's and Victoria's conversation after the dialogue had emerged.

The Importance of Responding

The development of the second phase of the Dialogical Investigations of Happenings of Change (DIHC) has greatly enhanced our understanding of dialogical processes in multi-actor discussions. It is not a method only to be used in dialogical therapy but in all conversations. A change in the very management of the affairs of everyone's life requires dialogue, whatever the approach guiding the action. One important point that has emerged is the importance of responding in dialogue. In multi-actor therapy, when responses are made, the responses are unlikely to ever match everything that is said. For example, therapists in their own responses or comments will pick and choose something, and these responses will have a major impact on how the dialogue progresses. In one couple therapy (Seikkula et al., 2011), a deeply depressed wife shared a number of health concerns and challenges she was facing at work, particularly with her supervisor. In talking about these, she said that her will to live had disappeared and when she said this, tears came to her eyes. One of the therapists turned to her spouse and asked how he had seen all this when he knew his spouse best. Her husband replied:

M: Well, I've tried to support Arja and... and discuss these things. I've tried to... sort of... to give my support to his work, to say that you can just try to manage your own work and your own affairs as best you can, and not think so much about what the boss is doing...

T: Yes,

M: That he should let things go in one ear and out the other. And I've been concerned, too, about her alcohol use... And... so... I've tried to discuss it with her. And now we've rented a house as a summer home.

This... in a way... has cheered her up a lot...

T: yes, hmh.

M: ...so we should have... we live in an apartment building and Arja... she gets isolated easily...

T: hmh.

M: ..home, not going out.

T: ymh.

M: But now I've noticed after 3 weeks in the country she's been much more active.

T: Was it this summer that you got the idea to rent this house?

The husband begins to describe his own concerns about his wife's situation, conflicts with his supervisor, managing work pressures, and Arja's excessive alcohol consumption. He also says that he has tried to support her. He then tells her that they have rented a house in the country as a summer place and that this seems to have cheered her up. Although he talks about a number of underlying problems, the therapists choose the theme of a new summer place. The choice, which at first seemed surprising, proved to be conducive to dialog, as it created an idea about resources in the midst of depression. Indeed, the therapists' response seemed to contribute to the creation of a transformative dialog.

Responses often emphasize that therapists are present at the moment and really hear what clients are saying in their voices, not from their own interest. Another important issue seems to be responding to the client's emotional experience. When clients describe life events and conflicts in the home, for example, the therapist's comment about paying attention to the emotional experience of the speaker makes room for dialogue.

Dialogue Is Built on Shared Experience

The new experience is therefore born of an increase in reflective capacity. In dialogical practice, everything happens in a shared development in which the therapists have a role and responsibility. But change cannot be initiated by some intervention from outside. For example, it is not a paradoxical comment by a therapist that creates change in the family system, but the experience of sharing together, where everyone can feel heard and accepted. The opportunity for reflective reflection often arises from life events, as was described in the experience of my friend's brother. A positive experience with his family enabled him to reflect on his own life and his own characteristics.

In difficult crises, we often need the help of others. There are many shortcuts to a shared dialogical experience. But unfortunately, there are also ways of talking that kill the shared experience that is already there.

References

Angus, L., Levitt, H., & Hardtke, K. (1999). The narrative process coding system: Research applications and implications for psychotherapy practice. *Journal of Clinical Psychology, 55*, 1255–1270.

Haarakangas, K. (1997). Voices of the treatment meeting. *Jyväskylä Studies in Education, Psychology and Social Research*, 130.

Linell, P. (1998). *Approaching dialogue: Talk, interaction and contexts in dialogical perspectives*. John Benjamins.

Luckman, T. (1990). Social communication, dialogue and conversation. In I. Markova & K. Foppa (Eds.), *The dynamics of dialogue* (pp. 45–61). Harvester.

Seikkula, J. (2002). Open dialogues with good and poor outcomes for psychotic crises: Examples from families with violence. *Journal of Marital and Family Therapy, 28*, 263–274.

Seikkula, J., & Olson, M. (2016). Therapists' responses for enhancing change through dialogue. In M. Borcsa & P. Rober (Eds.), *Research perspectives in couple therapy* (pp. 47–70). Springer.

Seikkula, J., Laitila, A., & Rober, P. (2011). Making sense of multifactor dialogues. *Journal of Marital and Family Therapy, 38*, 667–687. https://doi.org/10.1111/j.1752-0606.2011.00238.x

Seikkula, J., Karvonen, A., Kykyri, V. L., Penttonen, M., & Nyman-Salonen, P. (2018). The relational mind in couple therapy: A Bateson-inspired view of human life as an embodied stream. *Family Process, 57*(4), 855–866.

Vygotsky, L. (1935/1982). *Thought and language*. MIT Press.

Wertsch, J. V. (1991). *Voices of the mind: A sociocultural approach to mediated action*. Harvard University Press.

Chapter 9
Dialogical Science: Research in Real-Life Settings

The foundation of dialogical practice is strongly scientific, which is why the results have been so promising. This contributes to our understanding of the healing power of dialogical practice. Open Dialogues have developed hand in hand with systematic scientific research embedded in everyday clinical practice, in naturalistic research settings. The role of scientific research is to develop clinical practice in a broad sense—examining both treatment outcomes and dialogical processes. This is also an interesting phenomenon for research. In the development of dialogical practice, a new understanding has emerged regarding the role of science and research in the development of clinical practice in general and psychiatric care in particular. When I began designing the first study on dialogical practice in 1987, I had little idea about this. Over more than 35 years of research, a holistic research approach has developed its own phenomena and methods of implementation. In this chapter, I explore this phenomenon by giving many examples of how research has contributed Open Dialogues and dialogical practice, primarily in Western Lapland.

A Breakthrough in Psychotherapy Research

Research into Open Dialogue has not taken place in a vacuum but has developed in parallel with the revolution in psychotherapy research. When evidence-based medicine and its accompanying treatment guidelines began to make a real impact in the early 1990s, psychotherapists were reluctant to engage in research—especially regarding therapy effectiveness. This reluctance was evident in psychodynamic psychotherapy and family therapy. There was widespread concern that measuring psychotherapy outcomes through symptom ratings objectified clients and failed to reflect the essence of psychotherapy itself. Cognitive behavioral therapy (CBT), on the other hand, was from the beginning oriented towards short symptom-focused interventions, which were more readily studied using symptom ratings. The resistance to psychotherapy research has caused a lot of damage to the development of

J. Seikkula, *Why Dialogue Does Cure*,
https://doi.org/10.1007/978-3-031-91294-8_9

psychiatric care because it has given the floor to research that focus easily on inhuman treatment methods. The scientific rationale for treatment development was hijacked by research that was very one-sided and non-valid in terms of practical treatment development.

However, psychotherapy research has made substantial progress. Psychotherapy is widely recognized as an effective way of helping people if the results of therapy are measured by changes in psychological symptoms and experiences. Around 80% of clients benefited from therapy and 60% showed measurable improvement. In fact, no other method in any other medical specialty has achieved similar recovery. Psychotherapy tends to work quite quickly, with positive change beginning to occur within the first 6–8 sessions and within six months, 80% of the total treatment effect on symptoms is usually achieved (Wampold & Imel, 2015). The Helsinki Psychotherapy Project compared the differences between long-term psychodynamic individual therapy and short-term therapies. The latter produced equally good results, particularly in treating anxiety (Knekt et al., 2020). The Helsinki Project confirmed that psychotherapy is indeed very helpful.

Comparisons of different forms of psychotherapy have repeatedly found that there are no significant differences in outcomes (Wampold & Imel, 2015). When the factors influencing the psychotherapy outcomes were examined, it was found that the therapy methods themselves had very little influence on the outcome. Common factors to the different therapies were much more important. The most important of these is the relationship between therapist and client (Lambert & Ogles, 2004). Change during therapy seems to be more related to changes in the client's life than to psychotherapy itself. This whole reality is described by the concept of Common Factors in therapy. Thus, it is the nature of the working alliance, rather than the specific methods used by the therapist, that has the greatest impact on the therapy. Laska et al. (2014) published a meta-analysis to further define the Common Factors of different therapeutic approaches. They found that 54% of therapy outcome was related to the construction of a shared goal, empathic encounter in the therapeutic relationship, the therapeutic working alliance, positive feedback from therapists, therapists' authenticity, and the therapist's working characteristics in general. Only 1% of the variation in results was influenced by the specific therapeutic method used.

Although there has been less research in the effectiveness of family and couples therapy, studies have found similar results. Of course, family and couples therapy cannot be applied as widely as individual therapy—not everyone is in a relationship, and not all clients want to involve family members in the treatment However, family therapy has shown positive effects across a wide range of problems as part of other treatment (Sprenkle et al., 2009). In couples therapy, the effectiveness of Emotional Couples Therapy (ECT) in particular has been studied with good results. With a research team, we studied the effect of couples therapy in the treatment of major depression (Seikkula et al., 2013). We found that 69% of patients recovered from depression within 2 years and that the involvement of a spouse accelerated recovery.

In sum, psychotherapy research has indeed evolved rapidly and has provided an important understanding of the effectiveness of psychotherapy. From a dialogical perspective, it is particularly noteworthy that success is not driven by any particular method, but by the quality of interpersonal relationships. Dialogical therapy represents an extreme case in this respect, as it is concerned with good relationships and being heard. Psychotherapy research seems to support the importance of these values, as positive change has been found to be associated with a good working relationship in a variety of ways.

Naturalistic Research Meets the Reality of Care

Research is needed to develop dialogical practice. When beginning to develop our own practice, we need constant data to assess the effectiveness of the model of care and, in particular, to identify its problems. We can use all possible research methods. In fact, most often, the most valid research for a practice will come from the use of different methods in the same study. We obtain statistical information on changes in a group of clients treated and on the problems they encounter in their treatment. Simultaneously, we can see which specific cases are particularly informative for a more detailed qualitative analysis. The use of different research methods—a mixed methods approach—increases the reliability of the studies.

This kind of research can be called a naturalistic research design. Some have called it practice-based knowledge. The difference from an empirical controlled experiment is significant. In a naturalistic study, the treatment given to a patient is not controlled, for example, by ensuring that all patients receive exactly the same dose of psychotherapy. Instead, each treatment is tailored to the unique needs of each participant, using the most appropriate methods for each situation and each client. If the effectiveness of treatment is to be studied, comparisons are needed. Sometimes randomization can be used; sometimes information is on the outcomes of a group of patients treated at another site. This is called a quasi-experimental study design. We also need numerical descriptions of patients' experiences or to evaluate patients. Several traditional rating scales are also useful in naturalistic research. Since studies conducted by care facilities often do not have much external funding to hire researchers, the data to be evaluated can consist of objective events (sickness absence, disability leave, work attendance, readmission rates, number of days in hospital) and self-assessment scales.

In the field of psychotherapy research, methods have been extensively developed to assess the progress of psychotherapy processes by asking clients at each session both how they are doing and their assessment of the conversation. This provides information on the psychotherapeutic process in relation to the quality of the therapeutic collaboration experienced by the client. There are about twenty different types of questionnaires and, although they are largely designed to evaluate individual psychotherapy sessions, they can also be used to record the experiences of networks and families.

The research idea I have briefly described here is very useful for developing treatment. This is probably the main difference from the experimental research design. Whereas in a controlled trial, research is used only very narrowly to evaluate and compare treatment outcomes, in a naturalistic trial, all the information is used to develop the treatment itself.

The Role of Research in the Development of a Psychiatric Care in West Lapland

In developing care at Keropudas Hospital, and the Open Dialogue approach that emerged from its experience, we began, as early as the late 1980s, to study the practice in order to understand more about the processes of care and the results of the new family- and crisis-centered approach. Our confusing experiences of open therapy meetings were the impetus for starting this research. We had to begin investigating the phenomenon, as there was no previous research or textbooks on this kind of practice. At the same time, we also decided that systematic training of staff was needed to develop therapeutic skills for working with families. Research and training began to intertwine. We also made a cooperation agreement between Keropudas Hospital and the Department of Psychology at the University of Jyväskylä on a project to develop psychiatric care in Western Lapland. This was initiated by Jukka Aaltonen, Professor of Family Therapy at the University of Jyväskylä.

Over the decades, many studies have been carried out. It is not meaningful to go through them here, but I will give some examples of how research has been related to the development of practice in Western Lapland and what general conclusions we can draw about the linkage between research and the development of dialogical practice. It seems that psychiatric care in the Western Lapland Hospital District is one of the most researched care systems in the world. The Open Dialogue model of care is based on scientific research. In each new phase of change in the psychiatric organization, research was needed both to understand the new phenomena that emerged and to establish the effectiveness and efficiency of the new care practice that was initiated.

Open Dialogue was based on the needs-adapted approach developed in Finland, which aimed to integrate psychodynamic individual psychotherapy and systemic family therapy according to the unique needs of each patient and their family. As I mentioned earlier, the most decisive step towards a new approach to treatment was taken in 1984, when the hospital began to organize open therapy meetings. This practice continued for 11 years before, based on the findings of an extensive research project led by Professor Jukka Aaltonen, the comprehensive approach to care was named Open Dialogue (Aaltonen et al., 2011).

The studies have been carried out in two phases. Initially, the studies were directly related to the development of psychiatric care in Western Lapland. The second part of the research has been related in one way or another to understanding the different dimensions of dialogicity, both in Western Lapland and in psychotherapeutic processes more generally. Both of these parts have been essential for the development of the dialogical research tradition.

Hospital Admission: The Importance of the System of Boundary

The first major research project was carried out between 1988 and 1992. The aim of the study was to find out what happens at the first therapy meeting—the "admission meeting"—of a patient referred to hospital, when it was held before the decision to start hospital treatment was taken. A special crisis clinic had been set up at Keropudas Hospital for this purpose. The aim was to find out what happened at the first meeting and what factors influenced the decision to hospitalize. At that time, inviting families to discussions during the hospitalization of a family member was already commonplace, and we had realized that inviting families to open meetings created a particular way of interacting, which I called the boundary system. This research project resulted in the completion of both my own (Seikkula, 1991) and the doctoral theses of Chief Physician Jyrki Keränen (Keränen, 1992).

Study Design and Methods

All patients having a referral to hospital during a two-month period (September and October 1988) were included in the study. It was a "real-world" study because the aim was to follow the treatment process over 1 and 4 years in their daily care practice. The research methods used were simple statistical data on the patient's psychological status, Global Assessment Scale (GAS) scores, psychological tests (WAIS intelligence test, Rorschach personality test), psychiatric interviews, and assessment of the co-evolution of the team and the family using the Olson Circumplex Model method. A specific Clinical Rating Scale (CRS) was used to assess family interaction. Using the same method, I also developed a way to assess interactions within the treatment team using the same concepts as for family interactions. These by statistical tests to determine how much the team's activities resembled the family interaction system. In addition, case studies were used to illustrate the nature of co-evolution during admission meetings and throughout the treatment process.

Results

The decision to hospitalize or to continue treatment with home visits differed significantly based on the patient's previous treatment experience. A total of 70 patients were enrolled over the two-month study period. Of these, 14 were first-time referrals to hospital. Of these, only two were admitted, and 12 returned home after the first consultation, with care organized as home visits. The second group consisted of recurrent attenders (N = 26), of whom 14 were hospitalized and 12 returned home. This is a significantly lower number of home care decisions compared to the first-episode patients. The third group consisted of long-term patients (N = 32), of whom 26 entered the hospital and only six returned home directly. Their social network was so dependent on the care system that there was no possibility of finding resources for home care. At one-year follow-up, it was possible to conclude that the treatment decisions made at the first admission meeting were correct, as they did not need to be changed immediately. Jyrki Keränen compared the differences between the anamnestic admission interview by the doctor and the first discussion by the care team, and found that only the therapy meetings led by the team could focus attention on the patient's life and social network, whereas the admission interview by the doctor focused primarily on symptoms and treatment planning.

Conclusions

It is possible to find an alternative to hospital care if, in a therapy meeting held at the beginning of the crisis, the team, together with the family, can consider the life of the person in need of help in a broader sense, rather than just focusing on symptoms. It is easier to make a decision about home care in a first crisis than for a long-term patient. Overall, the need for hospital care could be resolved immediately for 40% of those referred. Also 15% of involuntary hospital referrals could be discharged at the first therapy meeting. The study taught us that it is important for the team to take into account the family's previous experience of care. In Western Lapland, this study was instrumental in closing the majority of hospital beds and shifting staff resources to mobile crisis intervention teams.

Qualitative Content Analysis: Creating the Open Dialogue

Professor Jukka Aaltonen initiated a research project on the dimensions of integrated community care (Aaltonen et al., 2011). The study was carried out between 1993 and 1995 with two main objectives. On the one hand, we wanted to understand more about the key elements of the new community care emphasizing crisis services, and on the other hand, we wanted to find out whether the new care model had affected the incidence of schizophrenia in the region. I was involved as a researcher.

Design and Methods

The study analyzed the medical records of all first-time admissions (N = 1918) from 1985 to 1994. Among these patients, we selected patients admitted for the first time for non-affective psychotic problems (N = 250) for further analysis. On the basis of the medical records, we aimed to follow the treatment of each patient for 2 years and to compare the treatment of those treated between 1985 and 1989 with that of those treated between 1990 and 1994. The idea was to identify the key elements of a new crisis-oriented and home-visit-based model of care. Qualitative content analysis allowed us to identify the key elements of the new model of care. In addition, we statistically analyzed the change in the incidence of non-affective psychotic problems over a ten-year period.

Results

Summarizing the qualitative content analysis, we found seven factors for optimal care. These are already listed in Chap. 1 (p. 20). In optimal process of care, the treatment started immediately in a therapy meeting within a day of contact, involved the family and other social networks of the person in the center of concern, selected the most appropriate treatment methods for the person, and the treatment team was available at all times, thus ensuring psychological continuity of treatment. In addition, the treatment process tolerated uncertainty by focusing the discussion at the meeting on creating dialogue and building shared understanding.

Once we summarized these key elements, we considered what we could call this new model of care. The idea of calling it Open Dialogue (Seikkula et al., 1995) emerged from the collective reflection.

Another important finding was that the incidence of schizophrenia had fallen rapidly during the development of the new treatment model. While in 1985 there were 33 new cases of schizophrenia per 100,000 population, in 1994 the figure was 7 per 100,000. Between 2003 and 2005, 10 years later, the incidence rate had fallen to around 2 per 100,000 inhabitants. The incidence of schizophrenia had therefore fallen by 90% over a period of 20 years (Seikkula et al., 2011a).

Conclusions

This research project was a crucial step in understanding more generally—not only in Western Lapland—the factors of family-centered crisis care. We also hypothesized that the decrease in the incidence of schizophrenia was related to the fact that in rapid crisis care, people with psychotic problems get help more quickly so that the period of untreated psychosis is shortened, and the problems do not have time to develop into the severity that schizophrenia has.

The Voices of the Therapy Meeting: A Dialogical Approach

Dialogue had at this stage become the main element of therapeutic activity. This development was initiated by my doctoral research and continued by Jukka Aaltonen's research project. As a next step, psychologist Kauko Haarakangas (1997), who had been involved in crisis work, studied the therapy meeting as a dialogical event.

Study Design and Methods

The study followed the live supervision discussions in three groups of the family therapy training in the Western Lapland Hospital District. In these, the team met with an experienced counsellor of the family in need. One case from each group was selected for further deep analysis. The researcher conducted a dialogue analysis of a specific therapy meeting.

Results

If the team and the family were able to create a co-evolving process, there was an opportunity to develop a more dialogical and resource-oriented approach as opposed to symptom-focused discussion. A particular understanding emerged from the study of the connection between the internal voices of the participants and the external voices that emerged between them. Kauko Haarakangas described this as a relationship between vertical (internal) and horizontal (social) polyphony. It also appeared that the training increased the therapists' ability to tolerate uncertainty.

Conclusions

This study contributed decisively to the understanding of the importance of listening in creating dialogue. The key to listening is to accept all voices. Polyphonic dialogue is a new form of family therapy and is different from other forms of therapy based on the centrality of language, such as narrative therapy. The study also confirmed the scientific nature of the psychotherapy training provided by the hospital district by analyzing family therapy dialogues. The findings were directly applicable to the further development of the training.

Integrated Treatment of Acute Psychosis: Three Open Dialogue Studies

The Western Lapland Hospital District was one of six research centers in the Finnish national API project (Integrated Treatment of Acute Psychosis). The study was conducted by STAKES in collaboration with the Universities of Turku and Jyväskylä. The total population of the study area was 600,000.

The key aim of the project was to develop outpatient care and increase knowledge about the role of neuroleptic medication in the psychosis treatment. In each research center—including Western Lapland—every first-time patient with psychosis was asked to participate in the study. Three of the six centers provided treatment in accordance with standard practice. The other three centers followed the need-adapted approach concept. With regard to medication, a new policy was created whereby neuroleptic medication was not started at the first appointment, but other active therapeutic methods were offered first and, if these were not sufficient, neuroleptic medication was started. Anxiolytic medication could be used for a short period to relieve the patient's anxiety or to treat insomnia. Psychotropic medication could be delayed for up to six weeks. In addition to these, in Western Lapland, we were also interested in gaining new information on how to avoid unnecessary hospitalizations.

The collection of survey data for the API project began in early April 1992 and ended at the end of December 1993. In the Western Lapland Hospital District, it was decided to continue a similar research design in another local research project from the beginning of 1994 until the end of March 1997. We called this project the Open Dialogue in Acute Psychosis (ODAP) study. About 10 years later, we conducted another ODAP II study to examine the persistence of treatment outcomes compared to the two earlier projects.

Study Design and Methods

All first-time non-affective psychosis (DSM-III-R diagnostic manual) sufferers aged 16–50 years were included. The persistence of diagnoses was 0.78 (Kappa = 0.453; p = 0.002). The main outcome variables were (1) variables describing the subjects at the beginning of treatment (psychiatric and social status, duration of untreated psychosis (DUP) defined as from symptom onset to first treatment intervention). As a second (2) component, we examined the variables of the treatment process (number of days and episodes of hospitalization, number of family therapy sessions, use of neuroleptic medication, and number of individual psychotherapy sessions). As treatment outcome variables proper (3), we examined the number of relapses (defined as readmission to hospital or the need to intensify ongoing treatment due to new symptoms), employment status, and the description of the patient's psychological state by the Brief Psychiatric Rating Scale (BPRS) questionnaire, the GAS scale, and one variable of the Strauss–Carpenter Rating Scale.

During the API and ODAP study periods, all the analyses were carried out by chief psychiatrist Birgitta Alakare and myself, so that we were not involved in the specific treatment processes analyzed. During the third ODAP II period, the research interviews were conducted by Birgitta Alakare together with an experienced nurse. All assessments were conducted at the beginning of treatment, and 2 and 5 years after the start of treatment. At the first treatment meeting, the family was asked for an assessment of the onset of psychotic behavior. In addition, Birgitta Alakare conducted an individual interview, which also included an assessment of the duration of untreated psychosis. The patient, their family, and all the staff who were involved in the process of care for them were invited to the follow-up interviews. This was to ensure that feedback from those who needed help was made available directly to those who provided care. This is an essential feature of a naturalistic research design, as the primary aim is to improve the care provided. The statistical analysis used Pearson's chi-square method and one-way Analysis of Variance (ANOVA) to compare the means of independent groups.

Results

One study report compared treatment outcomes for patients with schizophrenia with those of conventional care research center (Seikkula et al., 2003). In the comparison group, all patients had used neuroleptic medication, compared to 35% of patients in the Western Lapland API and ODAP groups (Table 9.1).

There were other significant differences in treatment processes as well. Patients in the API and ODAP groups had an average of 26 and 20 family meetings over 2 years, respectively, compared with an average of 9 in the control group. Patients in the comparison group spent almost ten times as many days in hospital (117 days) as patients in the ODAP group (14 days on average). In contrast, the use of individual psychotherapy as a treatment method was equal in all groups: about half of the patients had individual psychotherapy as part of their treatment.

The treatment outcomes were significantly different in the comparison group (see Table 9.2). In the comparison group, 74% of patients had relapsed, compared to 34% in the API group and 27% in the ODAP group. At the two-year follow-up,

Table 9.1 Use of neuroleptic medication in schizophrenia patients. Pairwise comparison

	API	ODAP	Comparison group	
	N = 22	N = 23	N = 14	P
Use of neuroleptics				
Started	8	8	14	***[a]
Continued	5	4	10	**[a]

[a] Difference between API and comparison group

Table 9.2 Outcomes of treatment for schizophrenia patients at two-year follow-up. Pairwise comparison

	API	ODAP	Comparison group	
	N = 22	N = 23	N = 14	P
Number of relapses	8	6	10	*[a]
Employment status				
Studying or working	13	15	3	
Unemployed jobseeker	1	6	3	
Disability pension	8	2	8	***[b]
Number of psychotic symptoms				
0–1	14	19	7	*[b]
2–4	6	4	7	

[a] Difference between API and comparison group
[b] Difference between ODAP and comparison group

Table 9.3 Historical comparison of API, ODAP 1, and ODAP 2 groups

	API	ODAP 1	ODAP 2
	1992–1993	1994–1997	2003–1005
Average age	26.6	26.8	20.6***
Duration of symptoms in months	19.6	10.2	11.4
Duration of psychotic symptoms	4.3	3.3	0.9***
Therapy meetings with family	22	16	26
Hospitalization days	26	18	14***

50% in the comparison group had visible psychotic problems, compared to 17% in the ODAP group. In the ODAP group, 91% had returned to active employment or were looking for work, compared to 43% in the comparison group.

In one study, a historical comparison was made between three different survey datasets in Western Lapland (Seikkula et al., 2011b) (see Table 9.3). This study included all non-affective psychotic patients, not only schizophrenia patients as described in the study above. During the first two study periods (API and ODAP 1), almost all patients asked to participate in the study were included. During the third study period (ODAP 2 from 2003 to 2005), the attrition rate was much higher. This difference seemed to reflect a change in the nature of psychotic problems in Western Lapland. Psychotic problems were no longer as common as they were 10 years ago. This seemed to be influenced by the fact that patients were seen, on average, as early as three weeks after the first symptoms appeared. The problems did not have enough time to develop into clearly detectable psychotic problems. This was also reflected in the significantly lower average age of the 2003–2005 participants. Patients in the ODAP 2 group who were treated at this time also had significantly fewer symptoms at the two-year follow-up. By this time, the crisis care system had been in place in Western Lapland for about 15 years, and it seems that people in the region learned to seek help earlier than before.

Predictors of Poor Treatment Outcomes

One of the main purposes of these "real-world" studies has always been to identify problematic situations in order to improve the quality of care. In one study, we included patients from the API and ODAP 1 study groups and compared patients with good and poor treatment outcomes (Seikkula, 2002). In total, 17 (22%) of the 78 patients were on disability pension or had visible psychotic problems. They were defined as the poor outcome group. They were more likely to have a poor social network and not to be in employment at the start of treatment. They were also more likely to have a diagnosis of schizophrenia and a longer duration of untreated psychosis. During the 2 years of treatment, they were more likely than others to be hospitalized and be on neuroleptic medication.

In another study (Seikkula, 2002), I investigated the differences between good and poor outcomes in relation to the quality of dialogue at the first therapy meetings (see Chap. 8). In the poor outcome group, the therapy meetings were mainly monologic, with the team failing to create a dialogue of shared reflection. In this group, the clients rarely initiated the content or manner of the discussion—or if they did, it did not become predominant in the sessions studied. In addition to these observations, the language domain in the topical episodes studied was mostly indicative: that is, they discussed concrete care-related issues, rather than the symbolic meaning of the expressions. It may be that, in a crisis involving strong emotions, the family has less opportunity for symbolic reflection on the different dimensions of the situation. It may also be that some families have fewer linguistic resources to begin with, so that the discussion is limited to expressions of concrete issues.

For the team, all of this becomes particularly challenging. On some occasions, the team was able to take initiatives in such a way that more dialogical dimensions and symbolic language began to enter the discussion. In one case, in the first therapy meeting, the team ignored the patient's own opening to start talking about his own violent behavior and "strange thoughts" and lost the opportunity to talk about these ever after. This case was described in more detail in Chap. 8. The team's attention was more on the client's account of what had happened than on what was happening at that moment in the conversation.

The Long-Term Effects of Open Dialogue

In Chap. 1, the results of a 19-year comparison between conventional care and Open Dialogue in Western Lapland were presented. This study confirmed that the tendency found at the two-year follow-up had continued in the same direction. The difference between Open Dialogue care in Western Lapland and the rest of Finland is staggering. When you add the fact that this is not an actual follow-up study of a treatment method, the results become even more interesting. After all, for the group Western Lapland, there is no control of the care after the first 2 years of treatment.

The study found, for example, that 40% had moved out of the area and were therefore likely to receive traditional treatment in a new crisis, where medication is suggested. Despite this, the differences between the groups are significant. The dialogical encounter they experienced almost 20 years ago seemed to still be having an impact on their lives.

Conclusions

Long-term follow-up showed that treatment results remained similar, and the difference compared to conventional treatment remained strikingly large. It is generally assumed in research that at long follow-up, the effect of the intervention can no longer be verified, because so many intervening variables enter people's lives. Contrary to this, the treatment experience of Open Dialogue seemed to retain its impact on people's lives for 19 years.

Based on this result, there should be no doubt about which treatment Finnish society should develop for the most difficult crises. The mere fact that in conventional care half of psychotic patients are still in treatment about 20 years after the start of treatment says a lot about the costs of conventional psychiatric care. Similarly, the high number of retirements is a good indication of the costs of conventional care.

From a research point of view, these results also confirm the high validity of the results of naturalistic "real-world" studies. The results obtained during the different study periods are consistent. In laboratory experimental settings, 20% of the efficacy of the treatment may be lost when the method studied is applied in the real world.

These results also call into question the drug-centered approach to the treatment of psychotic problems. Dialogue therapy does not focus on the elimination of patients' symptoms but seeks to consider the person as a whole and as part of a network of close relationships. In dialogical practice, the human mind is constructed in relationships, and so the person in crisis must be confronted in their relationships. But the results also show that this does not happen automatically, and that the treatment team needs to be properly trained. Even then, it is possible that the team may not be sensitive enough to hear the client's voice in order to create a healing dialogue, as was shown in the analysis of poor outcomes.

How to Understand the Results of Research?

The above section included excerpts from studies of Open Dialogue and dialogical practice. The aim has been to show how the research becomes part of the development of a system of care, helping to monitor both the successes and failures of the model so that it can be better adapted to meet the needs of the person in need. I have also been involved in other studies. For example, we developed a specific method for assessing the quality of dialogue in multi-actor therapeutic conversations (see Chap. 8). We also studied couples therapy in the treatment of major depression and found that involving the spouse in treatment speeds up recovery. We also found that there was a significant difference between the study centers in that depressed patients treated in the Open Dialogue treatment model in Western Lapland recovered better than patients treated in the other two study centers (Seikkula et al., 2013). In addition, there have been many interesting doctoral theses, including one on the internal dialogue of psychiatrists in the context of therapy meetings within the need-adapted approach (Borchers, 2014).

The studies have been significant in at least three different ways. First, they have described the results and problems of psychiatric care in general and of the Open Dialogue approach in Western Lapland in particular. This has been important throughout the process, especially at the beginning of the development, where we did not yet have an overall description of Open Dialogue. In the era of evidence-based medicine, these results have been vital in showing that serious alternatives to pathology- and symptom-centered treatment exist, and that it is possible to reduce the role of drug therapy in managing the most severe crises. The studies also showed that treatment outcomes improved when the starting point is meeting the person in their context and using drug treatment only as needed, based on individual requirements.

Second, the studies have been important for understanding and providing an overall picture of the foundations of Open Dialogue—and more broadly, of dialogical practice. Without research, the idea of Open Dialogue would not exist. Once this designation emerged from the conclusions of a study of qualitative content analysis of medical records, it has been possible to determine whether or not the care studied conforms to the Open Dialogue approach. For example, if there were no naturalistic studies of positive outcomes in the treatment of psychotic patients, the treatment guidelines of evidence-based medicine would almost certainly have rolled such radical new ideas.

Another vital source of information generated by the studies is the analysis of poor treatment outcomes. These analyses can help treatment teams to develop their own dialogical sensitivity to minimize failures. For example, a statistical analysis of selected dialogues in therapy meetings for patients with good and poor outcomes showed that those with poor outcomes appeared very different from the outset. The discussion was mostly indicative, focusing on practical issues related to care and daily life. Clients—both the person in need of help and their family members—were unable to take initiative either in choosing topics or shaping the way the discussion unfolded. It also appeared that the team's attention was focused more on what the client was telling than on being present in the moment. As a result, opportunities to discuss, for example, the client's psychotic experiences were often missed. This research finding has been very important for me in understanding how truly relevant it is to respond to what is happening in the here-and-now therapy conversations. I believe that without a systematic research design, such observations would have been missed or at the very least, only thought of. Now, they are registered in research reports and books and can be followed up in one's own clinical work.

Third, all the research I have conducted has been crucial in developing my understanding of treatment systems, the importance of family involvement, the nature of psychotic problems, and dialogical practice. Making similar observations in my own therapeutic work, supervision, or training situations would have remained much more vulnerable to outside influences so that it would not have been possible to open up a new paradigm of the human mind, of dialogical encounter and dialogical family-centered care.

In the process of conducting research, it is possible to take into account the importance of multiple factors acting simultaneously. When designing research, we make crucial choices. If we are designing a controlled trial, we need to control the treatment offered and make it a manual. In this case, we also need to limit the access of patients participating in the trial to other treatments and ensure that everyone receives the same amount of treatment. We must also choose data collection methods that guarantee the generalizability of the data and the neutrality of the researchers in relation to the patients and their problems. We face a wide range of ethical challenges. When designing such research designs, we create a certain psychological understanding of the subject of our research, and the risk of pathologizing the problems studied increases. Similarly, there is an increased risk of a straightforward cause-and-effect relationship approach, which simplifies complex phenomena. The comparison of differences between group means becomes the most important method for evaluating results.

In naturalistic studies, the thinking is radically different. Their aim is not to identify causal models to explain the results, but to study the phenomena in the approach described. Treatment is not controlled but must always be carried out according to the patient's needs. In this case, both the methods of treatment and the amount of treatment given can vary widely. In such a study, the treatment team is expected to participate in follow-up interviews and thus receive direct feedback on their work. The research methods are not pathologizing the problem, but more about the client's descriptions of their own experiences and direct observations from video recordings. These methods increase the external validity of the studies.

In all the studies I have carried out, one very important dimension has come true. I have never studied only the symptoms or changes in the symptoms of clients in care. I have always considered the care team as part of the interaction process. Even in the first study of the family–hospital interface, the interaction between the family and the team and their influence on each other was assessed. This has been the case right up to the most recent Relational Mind research project, which looked at the emergence of the human mind in the synchronization between therapists and clients. This is an essential part of a dialogical worldview. Knowledge is created in relationships and in the process of responding, and we cannot fully describe the object of study unless we consider all parties to the interaction.

The studies have demonstrated a high degree of external validity and reliability of the findings. For example, in the three different groups of studies of psychotic problems, no loss of treatment efficacy was observed, as is usually the case in controlled trials when a treatment model is applied to a practical treatment situation. This is a huge problem with experimental studies. Treatment guidelines may be written on the basis of studies that have shown that a drug relieves symptoms in 50% of patients. When that treatment is applied in actual practice, the effectiveness of the treatment may only be 30%, so 20% of the effectiveness of the treatment has been lost. Naturalistic research is able to control for this phenomenon of loss of efficacy. Unfortunately, experimental research designs do not take this into account. In Open Dialogue psychosis studies, three samples of studies achieved very similar results; this is very unique. To my knowledge, there are no other studies in which the same setup has been implemented in the same area three times in a row. I do not really know how the results could be even more reliable than that.

Criticism from Different Directions

Naturally, the studies have been criticized from various point of views. On the one hand, empirical research advocates argue that the results of the studies cannot be trusted because there is no comparison or control group. However, this is not true because comparison groups have been used, for example, in a quasi-experimental setting between two different research centers and in national register data. Others have criticized the fact that those who developed the treatment model were examining their own practice and that this makes the research data biased and not sufficiently objective. Freeman et al. (2019), in criticizing the evidence from the Open Dialogue studies, echoed these same points. They also argue that the studies lack an accurate treatment description model and a test of its reliability. This critique starts from the very idea that one should aim for experimental settings in which the treatment outcome obtained can be explained by a precisely described and controlled method. As I have said before, the basic idea behind Open Dialogue research is to generate information for the development of the treatment itself, not to determine the efficacy of exactly defined interventions. It is primarily a study to describe the treatment situation, not to explain the causes of the treatment outcome.

The criticisms of the research bias are in fact very important. It is essential to follow the tradition of scientific research in terms of the way data is collected and the methods of analysis. Since we have not been able to hire external researchers, using researchers from the same organization has been the only option. This is the case in general, since in about 80% of intervention studies, the developers of a treatment method are themselves the researchers of the intervention they have developed. It is important to use both assessment scales, for example on the development of symptoms, and objective data, for example on treatment use, relapse and disability allowances.

Criticism has also been leveled at the fact that the studies are only from Western Lapland, the place of origin of the approach. It is easy to agree with this criticism. We need research from just as many places as where dialogical practice is applied. Little by little, this research is already beginning to flow.

Some supporters of systemic family therapy and social constructionism criticize the use of statistical research. The use of symptom rating scales as a research method is often criticized because the scales objectify the subject. I agree that it is important to limit the use of assessment scales so that we do not think of them as describing a particular pathology per se, but rather the individual's experience of their life. I do not agree with the criticism of statistical research in general. We definitely need statistical comparative research, preferably combined with other research methods.

References

Aaltonen, J., Seikkula, J., & Lehtinen, K. (2011). Comprehensive open-dialogue approach I: Developing a comprehensive culture of need-adapted approach in a psychiatric public health catchment area the Western Lapland project. *Psychosis, 3*, 179–191.

Borchers, P. (2014). The need-adapted treatment of psychosis and the psychiatrist's inner dialogue. *Jyväskylä Studies in Education, Psychology and Social Research*, 507.

Freeman, A., Tribe, S., Stott, J., & Pilling, S. (2019). Open dialogue: A review of the evidence. *Psychiatric Services, 70*, 46–59. https://doi.org/10.1176/appi.ps.201800236

Haarakangas, K. (1997). Voices of the treatment meeting. *Jyväskylä Studies in Education, Psychology and Social Research*, 130.

Keränen, J. (1992). Selection for outpatient and inpatient care in a family-oriented psychiatric care system. *Jyväskylä Studies in Education, Psychology and Social Research*, 93.

Knekt, P., Lindfros, O., Heinonen, E., Maljanen, T., Virtala, E., & Härkänen, T. (2020). The effectiveness of three psychotherapies od different type and length in the treatment of patients suffering from anxiety disorder. In M. Ochs, M. Borcsa, & J. Schweitzer (Eds.), *Systemic research in individual, couple and family therapy and counseling* (pp. 349–366). Springer.

Lambert, M., & Ogles, B. (2004). The efficacy and effectiveness of psychotherapy. In M. Lambert (Ed.), *Bergin and Garfields's handbook of psychotherapy and behavioral change* (5th ed., pp. 139–193). Wiley.

Laska, K. M., Gurman, A. S., & Wampold, B. E. (2014). Expanding the lens of evidence-based practice in psychotherapy: A common factors perspective. *Psychotherapy, 51*(4), 467–481. https://doi.org/10.1037/a0034332

Seikkula, J. (1991). The family-hospital boundary system. [Family-hospital boundary system in the social network. English summary]. *Jyväskylä Studies in Education, Psychology and Social Research*, 80.

Seikkula, J. (2002). Open dialogues with good and poor outcomes for psychotic crises: Examples from families with violence. *Journal of Marital and Family Therapy, 28*, 263–274.

Seikkula, J., Aaltonen, J., Alakare, B., Haarakangas, K., Sutela, M., & Keränen, J. (1995). Treating psychosis by means of open dialogue. In S. Friedman (Ed.), *The reflecting team in action: Collaborative practice in family therapy*. Guilford Press.

Seikkula, J., Alakare, B., Aaltonen, J., Holma, J., Rasinkangas, A., & Lehtinen, V. (2003). Open dialogue approach: Treatment principles and preliminary results of a two-year follow-up on first episode schizophrenia. *Ethical Human Sciences and Services, 5*(3), 163–182.

Seikkula, J., Alakare, B., & Aaltonen, J. (2011a). The comprehensive open-dialogue approach (II). Long-term stability of acute psychosis outcomes in advanced community care: The Western Lapland project. *Psychosis, 3*, 192–204. https://doi.org/10.1080/17522439.2011.595819

Seikkula, J., Laitila, A., & Rober, P. (2011b). Making sense of multifactor dialogues. *Journal of Marital and Family Therapy, 38*, 667–687. https://doi.org/10.1111/j.1752-0606.2011.00238.x

Seikkula, J., Aaltonen, J., Kalla, O., Saarinen, P., & Tolvanen, A. (2013). Couple therapy in therapy for depression within a naturalistic setting in Finland: A two-year randomized trial. *Journal of Family Therapy, 34*, 281–302. https://doi.org/10.1111/j.1467-6427.2012.00592.x

Sprenkle, D., Davis, S., & Lebow, J. (2009). *Common factors in couple and family therapy. The overlooked foundation for effective practice*. Guilford.

Wampold, B., & Imel, Z. (2015). *The great psychotherapy debate: The evidence for what makes psychotherapy work* (2nd ed.). Routledge.

Chapter 10
Simple Steps to Develop Dialogical Skills to Be Present in the Moment

Having outlined above the factors that influence the effectiveness of dialogical practice, it is useful to summarize the basic premises of dialogical practice. At the outset, I noted my challenge in understanding the effectiveness of dialogical therapy practice. Based on the themes discussed, we can summarize guidelines for action to create a helpful dialogue. The aim is to find simple, enough practical and useable guidelines for any situation. Dialogue skills can really be learned. I was informed that radio journalists had been trained in dialogue. Listening to the programs of these radio journalists, I immediately noticed a big difference in the dialogue they had with the different people they interviewed. Conversations are no longer about exposing the other side to challenge, say, their political message, but more about finding the different dimensions of each issue to get to the bottom of things. At the same time, journalists are also capable of making critical comments, but now they contribute to a more nuanced understanding of each issue under discussion. These journalists seem to have adopted simple guidelines to generate dialogue.

When reading the guidelines of dialogue, it is good to remember that there are several paths to a good dialogue and not just one right option. But it is also good to remember that our actions can also easily prevent dialogue. The basic condition for a good dialogical encounter is that we learn to be present in the moment in order to respond in the best possible way. With simple guidelines like these, we can develop our own skills of being present:

1. Give priority to comments about this moment in this dialog—listen to what clients say.
2. Follow what your clients say and avoid making your own leading comments: for example, you can repeat what someone else said and ask them to tell you more.
3. Respond to expressions: responses are holistic, embodied experiences.
4. Pay equal attention to the different voices—don't forget the internal voices.
5. Listen to your own inner voice and bodily sensations.
6. Allow time for comments and reflective discussion among clinicians.
7. Formulate dialogical comments and speak in the first person.

J. Seikkula, *Why Dialogue Does Cure*,
https://doi.org/10.1007/978-3-031-91294-8_10

8. Take your time, with pauses and quiet moments to encourage dialogue.

Step 1: Dialogue Here and Now

In therapeutic conversations, as in conversation in general, we always make choices about what we respond to. The listener always "decides" what it is in the speaker's message at that moment that evokes his or her response. The word *decide* is in quotation marks because our decision is often made in seconds. If it is based on the response of the autonomic nervous system and the emotional experiences associated with it, then it is not always a conscious decision. But it can also be a decision that we make a considering a rational choice. This is usually the case, for example, in discussions between politicians or friends.

When the speaker's expression evokes a bodily response in us, it is good to try and broaden the field of dialogical response. The key to transformative dialogue seems to be to create a shared experience in which our responses emerge. Our responses emerge immediately, and attention to immediate experience seems best suited to attending to the speaker's experience in a broad, all-encompassing way. This experience is created implicitly rather than explicitly by framing our experience as a rational story. Implicit experience includes not only the spoken story but also the bodily emotional experience that accompanies it.

Considering the important information provided by the studies in dialogical therapy conversation, I have started to respond primarily to what happens in *this* conversation when each topic is discussed. The people who need help naturally want to talk about the things that have happened to them and how these have caused the crisis. They talk about something that happened in the past. But the dialogue is taking place in the moment. To respond to what they say is to respond to the past, as we only respond to what has been said. In contrast, the emotional experience that arises in a conversation is created in the here and now, and responding to it is the most important part of the dialogue. As I said in the example in Chap. 8, the speaker might begin to reflect on his or her own action here and now and *responding to that is more important than responding to what the client has told us.* In the example of the conversation described in that chapter, the team missed an opportunity to discuss the psychotic thoughts of a hospitalized patient when they did not respond to his reflection at that moment but instead focused their attention on the content of what he was telling.

I fully understand that this is not an easy task. In the case of the discussion presented, the team was concerned to find out what was happening at home when the concerned person said he had slapped his mother. They did nothing wrong, as finding out about the safety of those who have experienced violence is very essential. But this is the challenge of the art of dialogue: how to listen to the participant in the dialogue here and now as he or she talks about something emotionally charged? We easily get caught up in the details of extreme situations, which makes it difficult to meet emotionally the person who is telling us what happened at the moment.

Step 2: Follow What Clients Say and Avoid Making Your Own Leading Comments: For Example, You Can Repeat What Someone Else Says and Ask Them to Tell You More

A particular feature of dialogical conversations is that the facilitators of the conversation (e.g. the therapists) do not lead to particularly meaningful topics of discussion. The dialogue proceeds on the basis of the topics of discussion opened by the people who need help. This should be reflected at the start of the session in the facilitators' first lines, asking, for example, how the participants want to use this time together. Equally, the discussion can be opened with any other open question that allows the people who need help to start talking about what they feel is most relevant at that moment.

As in the example in Chap. 2, the facilitator's open question about how the participants would like to spend their time in a way that would be most useful to them encouraged the mother to talk about her concerns about her daughters and to reflect on what she had done wrong as a mother. An open question usually encourages talking about the most relevant issues. There is nothing to fear that participants want to talk off-topic and lead therapists to downside paths. Clients have a lot in their minds when they come to the discussion. Unless everyone has the opportunity to share what is in their minds, they may find themselves thinking about these things throughout the conversation and thus not fully participating in the dialogue.

In one family therapy process (see Chap. 6), the first question the person with the problem wanted to answer was how he would like to spend the time. He said that he had prepared himself by writing down the most important things. When the family was asked if it was okay for him to start here, everyone said yes. He began to read his notes, where the central theme was that shame was a big word in the family because he had always failed to meet his father's demands. He had written down several examples from his childhood. In one example, he told how his father was never satisfied with how tidy he kept his room. In his room, he would listen to father's footsteps approaching and he would try to hold up the door handle of his room violently to prevent his father from entering. Eventually, his strength gave out and his father entered the room and criticized him. I was very impressed with this story. I asked the father what came to mind, and he said he was surprised. He didn't want to be so hard on his children and hurt them. Then, I asked the client what he wanted to say, and he replied that maybe he wasn't so disappointed and ashamed after all. He seemed to back away from what he had said. I got a very strong feeling in my stomach about this, and I said that I did not really know how to react to his comment because I felt my stomach twisting. To this, he commented that it was the same as the feeling in his family. You never knew if you had done the right thing and enough because the messages from the father were so ambiguous. I felt that by giving space to start the conversation with his notes, we were immediately at the heart of the family interaction system.

Probably the biggest mistake in a therapy meeting is to start discussions by dealing with an agenda prepared in advance by clinicians. If we say at the outset that

"We are here to...," we are also saying that the issues on the minds of those who need help are secondary. This reduces their motivation for the natural reason that they become insecure about the importance of their own concerns. As already noted above, in dialogical therapy, there are no right or wrong issues, but a healing dialogue can arise on virtually any issue of importance to the client. What is more important is the emergence of dialogue, and with it, a shared experience of sharing. Because in the experience of sharing, those who need help gain more control over their own lives and become the authors of their own stories.

Most of the time in therapy sessions, I have a lot of different ideas and attempt to start telling the family or individual client how best to resolve the issue. A colleague once said that there is a lot of noise in the therapy conversation that makes it difficult to listen to the stories of the therapy clients. I often find that the noise comes from my mind. My way of managing the noise is to repeat what the client is saying in their words. This gives me both a little more time to savor what he is saying and to experience from the inside what it feels like to say those very words. In addition to this, I often find that the person telling the story is encouraged to say more when they realize that those words were not so dangerous and frightening after all.

These guidelines apply as much to a dialogue therapy session as to a therapy meeting. In a therapy meeting, not only the therapeutic issues are discussed, but also all plans and decisions related to the client's treatment. A good guideline is to set aside time at the end of each discussion for the clinician's treatment-related issues, but not at the beginning of the discussion.

Step 3: Respond to Expressions: Responses Are Holistic, Embodied Experiences

A dialogical community is created between the people present. So, it is essential that we try to engage everyone in the dialogue in their own way. It is an important responsibility of the facilitators to take everyone into account. This should be done as soon as possible and at the beginning of the discussion. My experience is that an open-ended opening question often immediately leads to what seem to be essential topics of discussion. It is good to encourage this. As in the therapy meeting in Chap. 2, the facilitator of the discussion immediately responded to the mother's concern and thus encouraged progress on the topic, so much so that she said she felt sadness in her stomach at what the mother was saying.

At the same time, it is important to consider everyone present, how they sit or stand, how they look, how they express openness or tension with their body postures, what their vocal balance is, and how they feel about the situation in general. It's good to give them space to talk at the beginning. If I oversee guiding the conversation, I might say to the first speaker, "What you are saying sounds very important. I would also like to hear what is in the hearts of the rest of you as you come into this conversation." We can go around in circle, where each person using their own vocal cords formulates a word, and as a result their tension is lowered and they become more open to listening to each other and engaging in the conversation later. I have had embarrassing experiences of someone in a conversation not being noticed at the start. In one case, I felt that we had a good dialogue and created a dialogical space for sharing. As we were finishing, a male participant asked to say something. What he said then brought out a very contrasting point of view. This experience was made more agonizing by the fact that he was a nurse colleague of mine whose concerns had not been addressed at the beginning of the conversation. So, he seemed to have sat throughout the discussion with this important point in mind and then, before the session ended, wanted to say it.

This example of poor response and poor consideration for all is very important to me because it reminds me that all participants contribute to the creation of an open space for sharing dialogue, for our colleagues as much as for our clients. Naturally, the focus is on the client's concerns, but the dialogue is no longer divided between the healthy and the sick; we are on an equal footing. This space for responding should be carefully nurtured in the dialogue. I try to take note of everything that happens and respond to everything. Of course, this is not possible, but it reflects an attitude of being present and attentive. It often happens, for example, that while I am talking to someone (e.g., my colleague), another participant comments on something. In this case, as a rule, I do not interrupt the ongoing conversation, but turn my gaze to the intervener and, nodding my head, say that I noticed him and later ask him what he wanted to say.

I may also interrupt an ongoing conversation if, for example, a person having psychotic experiences wants to say something. I see this as such an important opportunity to deal with previously unspoken experiences that I may respond immediately. I may also respond immediately to a young person who has been reluctant to talk about anything all along and then may, for example, talk over the other person to show his or her point of view.

Step 4: Pay Equal Attention to the Different Voices: Don't Forget the Internal Voices

Dialogue is more about how we talk than what we talk about. In our responses, we respond to the topic of conversation that the other person wants to talk about. But in my response commentary, I try to pay attention all the time to the prosodic side of speech and the messages of the speaker's body. In a dialogical conversation, I often sense in my body that the other person is beginning to move as he or she speaks. This can be manifested in a change in their volume, pitch, speech rhythm or breathing. Speech starts to slow down, they speak more softly, they seem to hesitate about what they want to say and take longer pauses. This is a dialogical gift because we are approaching something of the speaker's embodied experience for which there are not yet words or at least no ready narrative. So, we are approaching the most essential things.

How then do I respond by subtly opening that slammed gate? How do I respond so that I don't scare the speaker by fumbling something and get him to stop thinking about that topic? Virpi-Liisa Kykyri was a member of our research team, and her interest gave us a lot of new information about the importance of silence for dialogue. A co-authored article (Kykyri et al., 2017) gives the following example.

In this session, the client spoke of her disappointment at not being able to find a job despite her new qualification, despite having received good marks on her graduating certificate. She started talking about her painful and hurtful experiences with relatives and friends. She felt that she had been exploited by others for a long time. She named her father, sister, and close friend as people who often asked her for help but were not willing to help her in return. In particular, during her studies, the client had felt that she needed help and support but had not received it. Talking about these experiences, the client expressed her dissatisfaction with sad tears.

A: Mm (nods, wipes tears with hand)
T1: Before you didn't notice it and, well (.) the abuse just kept on (.)
A: Yes (wipes tears), go on…
T1: Mm…
A: I just need to be less—no—less involved so I can do well myself (nods).
T1: But is it so that now that you see that you have been used in those relationships, you feel bad about the invalidation and the lack of appreciation (.) that was not there before (points away from the client with his hand) or was that there too?
A: (Still wiping away tears) So that's what I was doing when I was performing.
T1: (Coughs) Yeah.

In this conversation, the client was very emotional, wiping tears from her cheeks with her hand. The therapist responded in a very soft tone of voice, showing that she was receiving and sharing the client's emotional experience. Earlier in the conversation, the client mentioned that at first, she had not noticed how she had been abused by her family and friends. Now, for the first time, she started to talk about it openly. The therapist repeated part of what she had said, referring to the feeling associated with the experience of abuse ("I felt bad"). The client confirmed this, to which the therapist responded with a sympathetic comment, "Mm." The client seemed to take this as an invitation to say more and to talk more about her experience.

When we were able to measure the autonomic nervous system responses, we found that the strong emotional experiences of the change in the prosody of speech are felt by both the speaker's body and the listener's body. When the therapist monitors the emotional state of the speaker by slowing down his or her own speech and lowering the volume and repeats something the client says, the client is encouraged to open up more to the new experience and form words for it. This experience can be very powerful.

In the context of our study, the client watched the described conversation episode with the researcher the next day. While watching it, the client was moved again and started crying. She said, "That's what I said. I remember saying something important, but I can't remember what it was." In a normal therapy session, we don't have the opportunity to rewatch important parts of the tape. It is important that we proceed at a very calm pace, and by repeating what the client is saying, we give space for the embodied experience to take root.

Step 5: Listen to Your Own Inner Voices and Body Sensations

In a shared dialogical space, we participate as therapists with our whole body. As discussed in Chap. 6, the autonomic nervous system connects us directly, that is, beyond our conscious decision, to our environment. We respond with the body's reactions; we cannot help but experience emotions. In a dialogical way of working, we also encourage therapists to live these emotional states. In our research on moments of change, we found that at the moment of a strong emotional experience, no change takes place, but the new thing is assimilated after the emotional experience. It is therefore very important to first give space to live the emotional experience and only then to start asking questions in which we ask those who need help to reflect on their own experience and its meaning.

This approach is very different from the systemic family therapy I adopted in the early 1980s. In the Milan systemic model, for example, therapists were told to avoid talking about feelings and to remain neutral. The aim was to steer the conversation towards actions and phenomena, not towards talking about feelings. In a dialogical approach to discussion, I tried to create a new emotional experience in which experiencing emotions and talking about them is central. This inevitably leads to the therapist's feeling they are an integral part of the shared experience because you cannot share the other person's feeling without feeling it yourself.

The dialogical way of working has many similarities with narrative therapy, but it also has clear differences of emphasis. Narrative family therapy has challenged the systemic perspective by emphasizing the importance of hearing all possible narratives, rather than therapists seeking only one and correct systemic description of the family. Combs and Freedman (2016, p. 213) described narrative therapy as follows:

"By relationships, we mean that our stories of ourselves and our possibilities would not exist outside of relationships; they have shaped our experiences with others and our feelings about how others perceive and react to us. We have been shaped by their responses and expectations. Our perceptions of what we can do are born out of memories of how people have responded to similar past events. In a sense, some people are present in the current event and in their understanding of others' expectations of me. We can hear, remember and learn stories of who we have been and who we are expected to be, and these stories are told in our relationships with others."

This view of humans is close to the one presented in this book. The dialogical approach adds more by embracing the embodied mind as part of the conversation, not just the stories described in language. The role of the moderator is also seen differently. While the narrative therapist engages the session with many different types of questions about the different voices of the participants, the dialogical therapist wants to participate in the emotional experiences that arise from telling these stories. A narrative therapist listening to the different stories may ask what surprised the narrator about this or that event. The clinician who emphasizes dialogue especially wants to experience the here-and-now feeling that arises from the telling of the event. Thus, the therapist may ask directly, "How do you feel about this?" Similarly, the therapist can share his or her own emotional experience by saying, for example, "I got very warm here in the pit of my stomach listening to you."

In dialogue, we need time to hear our own reactions. I have made it a habit to share something about my own bodily experiences in dialogue. This is not meant to be a specific new psychotherapeutic intervention, but more of an attempt to create space for myself to be more open about my own experiences. When I started doing this, I was very cautious and nervous about how clients would respond. To my surprise, I have not received any negative reactions to these comments about my own bodily experiences. Usually, I would say something simple like "When I listen to you, I feel the warmth here," and point to the top of my belly. But I can also say "I feel very excited here," pointing to the same place. It's very important for me to just say what I feel. It's not as if there's some therapeutic goal that makes it good to bring something up at this particular moment. When I feel tension in my stomach, it might be a response to some family experience that has not been put into words. My stomach is in sync with my clients.

Step 6: Allow Time for Comments between Clinicians

Discussions between professionals may have several meanings. In therapy meetings, all matters relating to helping the client are discussed openly in the presence of all. This involves formulating a care plan and making individual care decisions, such as starting a medication. In hundreds of follow-up interviews, I have heard how important this discussion is for families. They seem to be empowered by these discussions, so that they become more the authors of their own care, not just the recipients of different treatments. Robert Whitaker's book *Anatomy of an Epidemic* also interviews families who have experienced Open Dialogue treatment in Western Lapland. One of the families that was interviewed said that it is so important for all of them to hear what the staff think about them personally. They did not feel that it was so important for them to be informed about their family member's illness.

The second function of the conversation between employees is more about talking about the responses we get when we listen to our clients' concerns. Tom Andersen and his team originally called these reflective conversations. Tom's idea is that in a reflective conversation, the participant alternates between the positions of being the speaker and the listener. When we interview families, they are in the speaker's position, providing information and sharing their feelings and emotions. When I turn to my colleague and comment on how I have experienced what the clients have to say, their position changes to that of a listener. If we do this subtly enough, our conversations can create space for internal dialogue and reflection with clients. As in the couples therapy conversation in Chap. 6, clients can experience this very powerfully. After one network meeting, a friend of a young man with psychotic problems sent us a letter describing his experience of such a reflective discussion. He wrote:

"These new perspectives added to my own reflection and gave rise to some very stimulating new questions. We were all very open after the discussion to continue the dialogue among ourselves. Open Dialogue encourages ongoing discussion so that it starts to feel like a basic form of life, not just a method to achieve something. This is very empowering. (…) When professionals talked to each other and reflected on their interpretations in front of us, it added a huge amount to what we had been talking about from the beginning. (…) Through Open Dialogue, I have learned to explore issues rather than seek solutions. It has increased my compassion and patience in understanding all the issues related to my friend's psychosis."

In our research, we have found that reflective conversations are very powerful experiences for our clients. The experience of stress can be most intense at that moment. The experience of stress is good because it stimulates each person to listen intently, and then new learning is possible. But at the same time, it is very important not to cause too much stress, for example, by speaking in an offensive way or by criticizing. If clients feel they are being criticized, it triggers a defensive reaction in their autonomic nervous system, which prevents them from listening openly or learning new things.

When we developed the dialogues of the therapy meeting at Keropudas Hospital from the 1980s onwards, we learned to talk to each other very flexibly. I could comment on something at the beginning of the conversation and several times during the conversation, and we do not need to wait until the end of the discussion to have a reflective discussion. In a therapy meeting, we don't have a separate reflective team which only participates in the discussion by commenting on what they hear among themselves. In Open Dialogue therapy meetings, the clinicians are as much involved in interviewing the family as they are in reflective commentary with each other. The discussion between professionals also regulates their emotional experience and allows them to focus attention on issues that one of them might feel are important. The discussion between professionals can, therefore, have several functions in addition to its reflective function. When talking to each other, it is important to talk respectfully about family members. Similarly, it is important to speak only about one's own views, rather than attributing them as if they were truths. It is important to listen to the other's comments and to create a dialogue between us. Similarly, it is very important that when we talk, we turn and look at each other and not at the family. If, when we talk to each other, we look at family members, we are not allowing the family the space of a listener, where they can reflect on what they hear in their own internal dialogue. Then, at the end of each conversation, we ask the family what came to their minds as they listened to our conversation. This allows them both to correct our possible misconceptions and to form their first words after our conversation, thus storing this new experience in their bodily memory for further processing.

Step 7: Formulate Dialogical Comments, Speak in the "I" Form

Dialog is only possible between people. Mikhail Bakhtin (1984) distinguishes between two types of language, abstract and practical. In abstract language, we choose the words we use to describe some phenomena in life. For example, all theoretical descriptions fall into this category. Similarly, this book too is an example of abstract language. The author himself chooses his expressions rationally, according to the objectives he has created. Similarly, when discussing, for example, the nature of psychological problems, we use concepts of abstract language. This kind of discussion is often monologic. In it, the speaker has a desired goal which he wants to convey to the listener.

Abstract language uses a lot of attributes to describe phenomena. For example, all diagnoses are such attributes. The field of attributes has grown rapidly in everyday language. Today, we tend to express almost anything in terms of attributes. We can say that a patient is suffering from depression. Similarly, we can say someone is suffering from malaise, aggression, or irritability. It can be spoken about parenthood, short stature or long stature and so on. When we look for positive things, we can describe someone as cheerful or benevolent. This kind of vocabulary has also crept—or been triggered—into therapy work in many ways. With those words above, we can describe those in need of help as anxious, relationship-troubled, weepy, ambivalent, and out of control. The reader is free to add to this list indefinitely.

What's wrong with these words, someone may ask. The problem is that with such attributes, phenomena become, as it were, independent agents. We may imagine that they add to the objectivity or scientific quality of a phenomenon, but that is not what the words do. As a consequence, we then start looking for a reason for each attribute. What causes aggression, anxiety, depression or alcohol addiction? Life is full of different phenomena and explanations for them. These explanations are always simplistic and thus compelling for each person and can become a power trip against the other.

According to Bakhtin, the essence of dialogue is realized in practical language, in the use of language. All experience is created in expressions and in responding to them. In our endeavor to engage in dialog, we begin our expressions in such a way that they are always waiting for a response in order to be completed. The response of another participant in the conversation does not close and end the subject but opens up a new perspective. Instead of attributes, I speak about my experiences, my thoughts, and my feelings. I am very interested in your experiences in this matter, your thoughts and feelings. By participating in a conversation, I have denied myself the use of attributes. I will follow this rule absolutely in all situations of care. If someone in a therapy meeting says that a patient is suffering from schizophrenia, I try to talk about how he or she told me about experiencing these strange thoughts. If someone tries to find an explanation for the patient's behavior by saying it is due to schizophrenia, I do not engage in such a conversation, but I try to reflect on what happened to him or her just now that made him or her feel that he or she is being talked about in the soap opera in TV. The attributes that describe the phenomena do not cause anything, but people with difficult experiences can react in such a way that they start to hear voices, for example, or become depressed or anxious. In real life, all our bodily sensations, feelings, thoughts, and experiences are always responses to something, and these experiences are new initiatives waiting for the next responses.

The very nature of dialogue is to capture life in that infinitely rich and always unique form. As a therapist, I contribute to creating the most nuanced phenomenon possible by always speaking from my own point of view and not by attribution. My perspective is inevitably unique between different conversations and between different therapeutic processes.

Step 8: Take Your Time, with Pauses and Quiet Moments to Encourage Dialogue

In dialogue, we respond immediately to the initiative and utterance of the other person. Immediacy means that we sense the communication of the environment with our whole body, and through bodily action, we respond even before we become aware of what we have experienced and what we intend to respond to consciousness. Our body makes perceptions and begins to act without volitional control. Of course, within seconds, volitional control becomes part of this ever-flowing stream of responding. But as Quillman (2012) noted in their research, the client's autonomic nervous system is attuned to the prosodic qualities and bodily positions of the therapist's expression, that is, to the body's communication and not to what the therapist says.

In a multi-disciplinary therapy situation, many more dimensions of communication are involved. We are involved in a kind of dance where we are constantly adapting to each other through our body movements, changes in the volume and intensity of our voice and the rhythm of our speech. When a dialogical space of sharing emerges, the dialogue itself begins to guide its participants, not the participants themselves. In a space of sharing, our bodily experience calms down, and the need for argumentative, rapid discussion diminishes. This is often what happens in the conversations we have when we are highly aroused. Shared space also means that the rhythm of speech calms down, with longer pauses between words and between speeches. The need for each person to speak simultaneously with the other, for example, to correct this, is reduced. All this creates more opportunities for new bodily experiences and learning. One might think that a slower rhythm, including longer pauses and quiet moments, is one of the goals of dialogue.

Surprisingly, this dimension of dialogue does not seem to be a phenomenon of cultural differences. For years, I have had the opportunity to participate in dialogues in very different countries in the context of various training courses and seminars.

Finns are known around the world for their slow progress and silence, so this should come as no surprise to us. But a very similar process seems to be emerging in China, Japan, Italy, Spain, Germany, the United States, and South American countries. For example, the family that was presented in Chap. 2 often joked with their therapists about how strange it was that their way of talking became much calmer. This is probably a basic phenomenon of a dialogical encounter. When you have the space to feel your own experiences, it is also possible to begin to reflect on the painful issues in your own life in a safe enough way to learn new ways of working. To find new words and a new language for experiences that had not yet been narrated and thus manifested themselves, for example, as symptoms.

I often recommend to therapists to slow down the rhythm of talking and to be calm, to include quiet moments in their talking. There can be no dialogue without silence. In the silent moments, there is time for inner sensations and thoughts to take place during the speech, and thus for reflection to take place. Many have discovered the link between silence and dialogue. The Estonian composer Arvo Pärt has often been described as a master of silence. His impressive works, created on the basis of a few notes (he does not like to call himself a minimalist), are full of tonal variations, with both moments of very quiet sound and moments of total silence. A journalist interviewed him and was interested in these quiet or almost soundless moments. The journalist said that, for him, this music is very dialogical, influenced by those very moments of silence. Arvo Pärt liked this comment and added that for him, silence is so important because in the silent moment, he is closer to God. If you extend this beyond the religious experience, I can well agree with him. In dialogue, silence is so important because then we are in touch with the essence of life.

References

Bakhtin, M. (1984). *Problems of Dostoyevsky's poetics: Theory and history of literature* (Vol. 8). Manchester University Press.

Combs, G., & Freedman, J. (2016). Narrative therapy's relational understanding of identity. *Family Process, 55*, 214–224.

Kykyri, V. L., Karvonen, A., Wahlström, J., Kaartinen, J., Penttonen, M., & Seikkula, J. (2017). Soft prosody and embodied attunement in therapeutic interaction: A multimethod case study of a moment of change. *Journal of Constructivist Psychology, 30*(3), 211–234. https://doi.org/10.1080/10720537.2016.1183538

Quillman, T. (2012). Neuroscience and therapist self-disclosure: Deepening right brain to right brain communication between therapist and patient. *Clinical Social Work Journal, 40*, 1–9.

Chapter 11
Epilogue: Dialogue Is an Act of Love

While writing this book, I have had conversations with the voices of the people who have had a profound impact on my life. They are my interlocutors, my inner voices. I am very fortunate to have been able to enjoy a rich social and professional network. This network has given me the space to learn new things and grow into the clinician I am today. Some voices have influenced it in the past, but many voices are still influencing it today. I have worked a lot with Professor Tom Erik Arnkil, a pioneer of dialogical work. We also often have playful debates about how to illustrate the essence of dialogicity. For me, that essence is summed up in a statement by literary scholar David Patterson when he said:

> "Love is the power of life, its idea. There can be no dialogical relationship without love, just as there can be no love in isolation. Love is dialogical." (Patterson, 1988, p. 142)

Love is the driving force of life, the essence. This is also what I often hear in the feedback from families who have experienced the Open Dialogue process. One mother said that in the dialogue she learned to love her son again, with whom she had lost contact for over 8 years because of the child's violent arguments. Perhaps this also best sums up the answer to the fundamental question of this book: Why is dialogical practice so helpful? At its best, it crystallizes an act of love for us as practitioners, too. At the heart of it all is an unconditional respect for the other sufferer, and such respect can help bring about an encounter. In dialogical helping work, the focus is not on various therapeutic techniques, but on the basic values of life that take center stage. It is difficult to imagine a more important fundamental value than love and unconditional respect for others. Best of all, it is the most helpful and healing of all.

I dare to repeat this quote here at the end of the book, remembering Tom's comments on this. It is good to remember that we are always there as professionals, and our "act of love" is, on the one hand, very different from, say, a mother's love for her

J. Seikkula, *Why Dialogue Does Cure*,
https://doi.org/10.1007/978-3-031-91294-8_11

son or a spouse's love for each other. But dialogue is an act of love more than a method of treatment.

Reference

Patterson, D. (1988). *Literature and spirit: Essay on Bakhtin and his contemporaries*. The University Press of Kentucky.

Index

J. Seikkula, *Why Dialogue Does Cure*,
https://doi.org/10.1007/978-3-031-91294-8

MIX
Papier aus verantwortungsvollen Quellen
Paper from responsible sources
FSC® C105338

If you have any concerns about our products,
you can contact us on
ProductSafety@springernature.com

In case Publisher is established outside the EU,
the EU authorized representative is:
Springer Nature Customer Service Center GmbH
Europaplatz 3, 69115 Heidelberg, Germany

Printed by Libri Plureos GmbH
in Hamburg, Germany